KETO PASTA COOKBOOK

Keto Pasta Cookbook: 300 Tasty Recipes with Pasta, To Stay Healthy and Be Ketogenic Friendly. 21 Days Meal Plan Included.

Table of Contentrs

Introduction

Pasta is traditionally made of wheat flour, water, and eggs. Keto-friendly pasta recipes mostly require egg, little or no water, and flour alternative.

Flour alternatives are different from traditional flours because they don't have gluten. Gluten is what gives pasta a firm texture. Without it, pasta would become too mushy. For that reason, flour-based keto pasta recipes require thickening agents or stabilizers.

Common Ingredients:

Almond flour – Made with ground blanched almonds, almond flour is the most commonly used ingredient to replace regular high-carb flour in keto recipes. Compared to regular flour, it is richer in calories, fat, and protein.

Almond flour is available in health food stores, most supermarkets, and online retailers but you can also make your own using a food processor. When you buy or make almond flour, make sure that it's blanched and finely ground since larger particles can make the finished product less cohesive.

Coconut flour – Coconut flour is a fine, powdery, and dense flour that substitutes high-carb flour. It has less calories, fat, and protein compared with almond flour but is much richer in fiber.

Because coconut flour has a mild smell and taste of coconut, it's normally used in small amounts, way less than the amount of almond flour in a recipe. Another reason is that it may require more binders to keep the pasta together.

Coconut flour soaks up more liquid than other flours. To compensate for this, recipes with coconut flour require more liquids, such as water, oil, or eggs.

Xanthan gum – A popular food additive, xanthan gum is a powder that acts as a binding agent. It increases the thickness and prevents separation of food products. Although it's produced mainly with sugars, the carbohydrates in xanthan gum is 100% fiber, so it has zero net carbs.

Xanthan gum works like gluten, improving the dough's texture by making it sticky and gummy. Other ingredients, such as psyllium husk and gelatin powder, can substitute for xanthan gum but the resulting texture may not be that close to a normal flour dough.

Psyllium husk – This ingredient is commonly used as a dietary fiber supplement. In recipes, it acts as a thickener that binds ingredients together. Because it's an all-natural fiber, those who want a more natural approach to cooking can use psyllium husk as a replacement to xanthan gum.

When pasta noodles contain psyllium husk powder, discoloration can happen once they're cooked. Their color usually becomes grayish brown or purple.

Eggs and cheese – For flourless pasta, the main ingredients are eggs and cheese, particularly cream cheese and shredded mozzarella cheese. Recipes based on eggs and cheese usually don't require any binding agent. In fact, you can make pasta solely out of these two ingredients.

When a recipe calls for shredded mozzarella cheese, it's best to use mozzarella that's already shredded at the store instead of shredding the cheese yourself.

Whey isolate or protein powder – The main reason for using whey isolate as a flour substitute in keto pasta recipes isn't just to make your food more protein-rich. Whey isolate actually works like gluten, binding all the ingredients together and improves the consistency of dough.

One specific type of protein powder is micellar casein. Some observe that this slow-digesting dairy protein can make dough thicker.

Pork rinds – Although this ingredient isn't commonly used in making low-carb pasta, pork rinds make a good flour substitute. They are high in protein and fat and contain no carbohydrates.

Glucomannan powder – This zero-calorie ingredient is derived from the root of konjac plant, the same plant that is used to make shirataki or miracle noodles. Also known as konjac powder, it acts as a thickening agent.

Soy flour – Another low-carb flour alternative, soy flour is made from ground soybeans. It is richer in protein than other keto flours and a good source of fiber. Like coconut flour, it easily absorbs liquid so recipes with soy flour usually require water.

Oat fiber – Made from the hull of oat, this ingredient is an insoluble fiber with a texture similar to whole-wheat flour. It acts as a binding agent together with almond, coconut, and other low-carb flours.

Vital wheat gluten – This ingredient is made from wheat flour that's almost pure gluten with minimal starch. It's rich in protein but low in carbs. Adding a small amount of vital wheat gluten to a recipe improves the elasticity of the dough, making it close to the real thing.

Chapter 1. How To Choose Keto Pasta

We understand if you cannot spend half your time in the kitchen, whipping up a MasterChef dish from scratch. That is why many food producers have created pre-packaged goods, canned and dried goods. Fresh is best but when in a hurry, it is best to opt for the simplest solution.

When it comes to pasta there are a wide variety of pastas to make and of course an array of dried pastas to choose from, all boasting an assortment of shapes and colors.

Each pasta is actually made with the sauce in mind, they are created to ensure that you as the person enjoying the meal revels in all the tastes and textures that there are without comprising the pasta or the sauce.

Let us help you to understand the very basics of which pasta to use and what sauce to use when creating your next pasta feast.

1. Top Tips

1. Choose pasta made from durum wheat whenever you can.

2. If you can, buy a packet of pasta that was imported from Italy.

3. Pasta is either made using durum wheat flour and water or durum wheat flour and egg. Neither is better than the other. It is suggested that sauces that are rich with butter and cream are served with egg-based pastas. Sauces that are oil-based are generally served with the regular made pasta.

4. Consider the following, saucey toppings are best suited to long, ribbon like pasta such as linguine or spaghetti. Chunkier sauces with more textures are best suited to short based pasta such as penne or rigatoni.

5. These are guidelines to help aid you in serving a hearty dish that you can be proud of. In the end, cooking comes from the heart, do what you feel is best or what you and your family enjoy.

2. Short Pastas

Keep one thing in mind when cooking short pasta, and that is it should be that the size of the pasta and ingredients complement one another. The thicker, chunkier the sauce the bigger or larger the groove and hollow of the pasta should be to allow for an even, mouthful of both pasta and sauce.

Short pasta shapes work well in soups, salads, stews, baked and with meatier, cheesy sauces. All short pastas can be substituted with one another.

Pasta with grooves or spirals are great for catching sauce in them. It is best to always add your pasta to the sauce and give it a good stir so that the sauce can travel into these pockets, guaranteeing you a delicious bite every time.

Risoni, wheeled pasta, star-shaped and small, shelled pastas are perfect for soups when you are required to boil the pasta in the sauce.

Farfalla and spiral pasta are wonderful for salads as the light dressings used such as olive oils, vinegars and lemon juice are held within the groves and they make for a pretty dish to place upon a table come serving time.

Short pastas such as cannelloni, are boiled, stuffed then baked.

Some short pasta varieties to try and include in your cooking are:

- Cannelloni

- Conchiglie

- Farfalle

- Fusilli

- Gemelli

- Gnocchetti

- Lasagna

- Macaroni

- Orecchiette

- Penne

- Rigatoni

- Risoni

- Spiral Pasta

- Star-shaped Pasta

- Vermicelli

- Wheel-shaped Pasta

3. Long Pastas

The same variety of shapes and sizes exist in reference to long pasta too. Often long and thin shaped pastas are reserved for sauces that easily glide over them such as oil based ones. The concept is that when scooping the pasta up to eat, the sauce clings to the strands as you eat. It is best to use a fork when planning on eating long stranded pastas.

Oil-based, tomato-based and cheese sauces work well with long, ribboned pastas. Seafood pasta dishes are commonly served with long, thin stranded pasta such as spaghetti or capellini.

For long stranded pasta which is wider such as pappardelle meat sauces and ragus compliment this pasta superbly.

A simple rule to apply when partnering sauces and long pastas is, "Will the sauce cling to the pasta when eaten with a fork?"

Some long pasta varieties to try and include in your cooking are:

- Bucatini

- Capellini/ Angel's Hair

- Fettuccini

- Linguini

- Parpadelle

- Spaghetti

- Tagliatelle

- Ziti

4. Fresh Pastas

Some delis and supermarkets have specialty aisles where you may come across freshly made pastas. They also carry an array of colors, shapes and sizes. It is important to remember that fresh pasta cooks far faster than dried.

Filled short pasta such as ravioli and tortellini have already been stuffed with a unique filling such as pancetta, butternut, nuts, herbs and cheeses and are traditionally boiled before adding a sauce or a dash of melted butter. The sauces recommended for these are mild and thin so as not to conflict with the stuffing used.

Gnocchi goes just as well with thin based sauces and is also delicious when baked in a cheese sauce.

Some fresh pasta varieties to try and include in your cooking are:

- Gnocchi

- Ravioli

- Tortellini

5. Flavored and Colored Pastas

The most common color of pasta is a creamy white or pale yellow and that is because of the flour and of course the eggs used to make the pasta.

Pasta does however come a selection of different colors, all which contribute to added flavor and texture. Some pastas to look out for include:

Pasta Verde - This is known as green pasta. During the process of making the dough, herbs or the juice of spinach are added to give it its green colour. It is not uncommon to find green lasagna or tagliatelle at your supermarket.

Black Pasta - This is pasta that has been dyed black using the ink from a squid. This type of pasta if obviously best used when making seafood dishes.

Orange Pasta - Orange colored pastas are made from carrot juice.

Red Pasta - Red pasta is made using beetroot juice.

Bright Yellow Pasta - Brightly colored yellow pastas are made using saffron during the production process.

Chapter 2. Low Carb Pasta

6. Zucchini Vegan Bacon Lasagna

Preparation Time: 15 minutes
Cooking Time: 40 minutes
Servings: 4

Ingredients:

4 large yellow zucchinis

Salt and black pepper to taste

1 tbsp lard

½ lb vegan bacon

1 tsp garlic powder

1 tsp onion powder

2 tbsp coconut flour

1 ½ cup grated mozzarella cheese

1/3 cup cheddar cheese

2 cups crumbled ricotta cheese

1 large egg

2 cups unsweetened marinara sauce

1 tbsp Italian herb seasoning

¼ tsp red chili flakes

¼ cup fresh basil leaves

Directions:

Preheat the oven to 375 F and grease a 9 x 9-inch baking dish with cooking spray. Set aside.

Slice the zucchini into ¼ -inch strips, arrange on a flat surface and sprinkle generously with salt. Set aside to release liquid for 5 to 10 minutes. Pat dry with a paper towel and set aside.

Melt the lard in a large skillet over medium heat and add the vegan bacon. Cook until browned, 10 minutes. Set aside to cool.

In a medium bowl, evenly combine the garlic powder, onion powder, coconut flour, salt, black pepper, mozzarella cheese, half of the cheddar cheese, ricotta cheese, and egg. Set aside.

Add the Italian herb seasoning and red chili flakes to the marinara sauce and mix. Set aside.

Make a single layer of the zucchini in the baking dish; spread a quarter of the egg mixture on top, and a quarter of the marinara sauce. Repeat the layering process and sprinkle the top with the remaining cheddar cheese.

Bake in the oven for 30 minutes or until golden brown on top.

Remove the dish from the oven, allow cooling for 5 to 10 minutes, garnish with the basil leaves, slice and serve.

Nutrition:

Calories:417 , Total Fat: 36.4g, Saturated Fat: 15.9g, Total Carbs: 4g, Dietary Fiber:0g, Sugar: 1g, Protein20: g, Sodium: 525mg

7. Parsley-Lime Pasta

Preparation Time: 20 minutes
Servings: 4

Ingredients:

2 tbsp butter

1 lb tempeh, chopped

4 garlic cloves, minced

1 pinch red chili flakes

¼ cup white wine

1 lime, zested and juiced

3 medium zucchinis, spiralized

Salt and black pepper to taste

2 tbsp chopped parsley

1 cup grated parmesan cheese for topping

Directions:

Melt the butter in a large skillet and cook in the tempeh until golden brown.

Flip and stir in the garlic and red chili flakes. Cook further for 1 minute; transfer to a plate and set aside.

Pour the wine and lime juice into the skillet, and cook until reduced by a quarter. Meanwhile, stir to deglaze the bottom of the pot.

Mix in the zucchinis, lime zest, tempeh and parsley. Season with salt and black pepper, and toss everything well. Cook until the zucchinis is slightly tender for 2 minutes.

Dish the food onto serving plates and top generously with the parmesan cheese.

Nutrition:

Calories: 326, Total Fat: 24.9g, Saturated Fat:12.9 g, Total Carbs: 6 g, Dietary Fiber:1g, Sugar: 4g, Protein: 20g, Sodium: 568mg

8. Creamy Garlic Mushrooms With Angel Hair Shirataki

Preparation Time: 25 minutes

Servings: 4

Ingredients:

For the mushroom sauce:

1 tbsp olive oil

1 lb chopped mushrooms

Salt and black pepper to taste

2 tbsp unsalted butter

6 garlic cloves, minced

½ cup dry white wine

1 ½ cups coconut cream

½ cup grated parmesan cheese

2 tbsp chopped fresh parsley

For the angel hair shirataki:

2 (8 oz) packs angel hair shirataki noodles

Salt to season

Directions:

For the mushroom sauce:

Heat the olive oil in a large skillet, season the mushroom with salt and black pepper, and cook in the oil until softened, 5 minutes. Transfer to a plate and set aside.

Melt the butter in the skillet and sauté the garlic until fragrant. Stir in the white wine and cook until reduced by half, meanwhile, scraping the bottom of the pan to deglaze.

Reduce the heat to low and stir in the coconut cream. Allow simmering for 1 minute and stir in the parmesan cheese to melt.

Return the mushroom to the sauce and sprinkle the parsley on top. Adjust the taste with salt and black pepper, if needed.

For the angel hair shirataki:

Bring 2 cups of water to a boil in a medium pot over medium heat.

Strain the shirataki pasta through a colander and rinse very well under hot running water.

Allow proper draining and pour the shirataki pasta into the boiling water. Cook for 3 minutes and strain again.

Place a dry skillet over medium heat and stir-fry the shirataki pasta until visibly dry and makes a squeaky sound when stirred, 1 to 2 minutes.

Season with salt and plate.

Top the shirataki pasta with the mushroom sauce and serve warm.

Nutrition:

Calories: , Total Fat: g, Saturated Fat: g, Total Carbs: g, Dietary Fiber:g, Sugar: g, Protein: g, Sodium: mg

Nutrition:

Calories:89 , Total Fat:6.4 g, Saturated Fat:1.5 g, Total Carbs: 2g, Dietary Fiber:0g, Sugar:1g, Protein:6 g, Sodium: 406mg

9. Coconut Tofu Zucchini Bake

Preparation Time: 40 minutes
Servings: 4

Ingredients:

1 tbsp butter

1 cup green beans, chopped

1 bunch asparagus, trimmed and cut into 1-inch pieces

2 tbsp arrowroot starch

2 cups coconut milk

4 medium zucchinis, spiralized

1 cup grated parmesan cheese

1 (15 oz) firm tofu, pressed and sliced

Salt and black pepper to taste

Directions:

Preheat the oven to 380 F.

Melt the butter in a medium skillet and sauté the green beans and asparagus until softened, about 5 minutes. Set aside.

In a medium saucepan, mix the arrowroot starch with the coconut milk. Bring to a boil over medium heat with frequent stirring until thickened, 3 minutes. Stir in half of the parmesan cheese until melted.

Mix in the green beans, asparagus, zucchinis and tofu. Season with salt and black pepper.

Transfer the mixture to a baking dish and cover the top with the remaining parmesan cheese.

Bake in the oven until the cheese melts and golden on top, 20 minutes.

Remove the food from the oven and serve warm.

Nutrition:

Calories: 492, Total Fat:26.8 g, Saturated Fat: 12.6g, Total Carbs: 14g, Dietary Fiber:4g, Sugar: 8g, Protein: 50g, Sodium: 1668mg

10. Creamy Seitan Shirataki Fettucine

Preparation Time: 35 minutes

Servings: 4

Ingredients:

For the shirataki fettuccine:

2 (8 oz) packs shirataki fettuccine

For the creamy seitan sauce:

5 tbsp butter

4 seitan slabs, cut into 2-inch cubes

Salt and black pepper to taste

3 garlic cloves, minced

1 ¼ cups coconut cream

½ cup dry white wine

1 tsp grated lemon zest

1 cup baby spinach

Lemon wedges for garnishing

Directions:

For the shirataki fettuccine:

Boil 2 cups of water in a medium pot over medium heat.

Strain the shirataki pasta through a colander and rinse very well under hot running water.

Allow proper draining and pour the shirataki pasta into the boiling water. Cook for 3 minutes and strain again.

Place a dry skillet over medium heat and stir-fry the shirataki pasta until visibly dry, and makes a squeaky sound when stirred, 1 to 2 minutes. Take off the heat and set aside.

For the seitan sauce:

Melt half of the butter in a large skillet; season the seitan with salt, black pepper, and cook in the butter until golden brown on all sides and flaky within, 8 minutes. Transfer to a plate and set aside.

Add the remaining butter to the skillet to melt and stir in the garlic. Cook until fragrant, 1 minute.

Mix in the coconut cream, white wine, lemon zest, salt, and black pepper. Allow boiling over low heat until the sauce thickens, 5 minutes.

Stir in the spinach, allow wilting for 2 minutes and stir in the shirataki fettuccine and seitan until well-coated in the sauce. Adjust the taste with salt and black pepper.

Dish the food and garnish with the lemon wedges. Serve warm.

Nutrition:

Calories: 720, Total Fat: 56.5g, Saturated Fat: 27.2g, Total Carbs: 17 g, Dietary Fiber:3g, Sugar: 7g, Protein: 37g, Sodium:1764 mg

11. Tofu And Spinach Lasagna With Red Sauce

Prep Time: 20minutes
Cooking Time: 45minutes
Servings: 4

Ingredients:

2 tbsp butter

1 white onion, chopped

1 garlic clove, minced

2 ½ cups crumbled tofu

3 tbsp tomato paste

½ tbsp dried oregano

1 tsp salt

¼ tsp ground black pepper

½ cup water

1 cup baby spinach

For the low-carb pasta:

Flax egg: 8 tbsp flax seed powder + 1 ½ cups water

1 ½ cup dairy-free cashew cream

1 tsp salt

5 tbsp psyllium husk powder

For topping:

2 cups coconut cream

5 oz. shredded mozzarella cheese

2 oz. grated tofu cheese

½ tsp salt

¼ tsp ground black pepper

½ cup fresh parsley, finely chopped

Directions:

Melt the butter in a medium pot over medium heat. Then, add the white onion and garlic, and sauté until fragrant and soft, about 3 minutes.

Stir in the tofu and cook until brown. Mix in the tomato paste, oregano, salt, and black pepper.

Pour the water into the pot, stir, and simmer the Ingredients until most of the liquid has evaporated.

While cooking the sauce, make the lasagna sheets. Preheat the oven to 300 F and mix the flax seed powder with the water in a medium bowl to make flax egg. Allow sitting to thicken for 5 minutes.

Combine the flax egg with the cashew cream and salt. Add the psyllium husk powder a bit at a time while whisking and allow the mixture to sit for a few more minutes.

Line a baking sheet with parchment paper and spread the mixture in. Cover with another parchment paper and use a rolling pin to flatten the dough into the sheet.

Bake the batter in the oven for 10 to 12 minutes, remove after, take off the parchment papers, and slice the pasta into sheets that fit your baking dish.

In a bowl, combine the coconut cream and two-thirds of the mozzarella cheese. Fetch out 2 tablespoons of the mixture and reserve.

Mix in the tofu cheese, salt, black pepper, and parsley. Set aside.

Grease your baking dish with cooking spray and lay in one-third of the pasta sheet; spread half of the tomato sauce on top, add another one-third set of the pasta sheets, the remaining tomato sauce and the rest of the pasta sheets.

Grease your baking dish with cooking spray, layer a single line of pasta in the dish, spread with some tomato sauce, 1/3 of the spinach, and ¼ of the coconut cream mixture. Season with salt and black pepper as desired.

Repeat layering the Ingredients twice in the same manner making sure to top the final layer with the coconut cream mixture and the reserved cashew cream.

Bake in the oven for 30 minutes at 400 F or until the lasagna has a beautiful brown surface.

Remove the dish; allow cooling for a few minutes, and slice.

Serve the lasagna with a baby green salad.

Nutrition:

Calories: 487, Total Fat:45.3g, Saturated Fat:34.2g, Total Carbs: 13g, Dietary Fiber:3g, Sugar: 2g, Protein: 14g, Sodium:459 mg

12. Zoodle Bolognese

Prep Time: 10minutes
Cooking Time: 35minutes
Servings: 4

Ingredients:

For the Bolognese sauce:

3 oz. olive oil

1 white onion, chopped

1 garlic clove, minced

3 oz. celery, chopped

3 cups crumbled tofu

2 tbsp tomato paste

1 ½ cups crushed tomatoes

1 tsp salt

¼ tsp black pepper

1 tbsp dried basil

1 tbsp Worcestershire sauce

Water as needed

For the zoodles:

1 lb zucchinis

2 tbsp butter

Salt and black pepper to taste

Directions:

Pour the olive oil into a saucepan and heat over medium heat. When no longer shimmering, add the onion, garlic, and celery. Sauté for 3 minutes or until the onions are soft and the carrots caramelized.

Pour in the tofu, tomato paste, tomatoes, salt, black pepper, basil, and Worcestershire sauce. Stir and cook for 15 minutes, or simmer for 30 minutes.

Mix in some water if the mixture is too thick and simmer further for 20 minutes.

While the sauce cooks, make the zoodles. Run the zucchini through a spiralizer to form noodles.

Melt the butter in a skillet over medium heat and toss the zoodles quickly in the butter, about 1 minute only.

Season with salt and black pepper.

Nutrition:

Calories: ,239 Total Fat:14.7g, Saturated Fat:8.1g, Total Carbs: 14g, Dietary Fiber:1g, Sugar:7 g, Protein: 13g, Sodium: 530mg

13. Creamy Mushrooms With Shirataki

Preparation Time: 25 minutes

Servings: 4

Ingredients:

For the angel hair shirataki:

2 (8 oz) packs angel hair shirataki

For the creamy mushrooms:

4 tbsp olive oil

1 lb sliced cremini mushrooms

3 shallots, finely chopped

6 garlic cloves, minced

2 tsp red chili flakes

¼ cup white wine

½ cup vegetable stock

1 ½ cups coconut cream

2 tbsp chopped fresh parsley

Salt and black pepper to taste

Directions:

For the angel hair shirataki:

Bring 2 cups of water to a boil in a medium pot over medium heat.

Strain the shirataki pasta through a colander and rinse very well under hot running water.

Drain properly and transfer the shirataki pasta into the boiling water. Cook for 3 minutes and strain again.

Place a large dry skillet over medium heat and stir-fry the shirataki pasta until visibly dry, 1 to 2 minutes. Take off the heat and set aside.

For the creamy mushrooms:

Heat the olive oil in a large skillet and sauté the mushrooms, shallots, garlic, and chili flakes until softened and fragrant, 3 minutes.

Mix in the white wine and vegetable stock. Allow boiling and whisk in the remaining butter and then the coconut cream.

Taste the sauce and adjust the taste with salt, black pepper, and mix in the parsley.

Pour in the shirataki pasta, mussels and toss well in the sauce.

Serve afterwards.

Nutrition:

Calories:673 , Total Fat:58.8g, Saturated Fat:36.3g, Total Carbs: 16g, Dietary Fiber:7, Sugar:2 g, Protein: 26g, Sodium:760 mg

14. Tempeh Alfredo Squash Spaghetti

Preparation Time: 1 hour and 20 minutes

Servings: 4

Ingredients:

For the pasta:

2 medium spaghetti squashes, halved

2 tbsp olive oil

For the sauce:

2 tbsp butter

1 lb tempeh, crumbled

½ tsp garlic powder

Salt and black pepper to taste

1 tsp arrowroot starch

1 ½ cups coconut cream

A pinch of nutmeg

1/3 cup finely grated parmesan cheese

1/3 cup finely grated tempeh mozzarella cheese

Directions:

Preheat the oven to 375 F and line a baking dish with foil. Set aside.

Season the squash with the olive oil, salt, and black pepper. Place the squash on the baking dish, open side up and roast for 45 to 50 minutes until the squash is tender.

When ready, remove the squash from the oven, allow cooling and use two forks to shred the inner part of the noodles. Set aside.

Melt the butter in a medium pot, add the tempeh, garlic powder, salt, and black pepper, cook until brown, 10 minutes.

Stir in the arrowroot starch, coconut cream, and nutmeg. Cook until the sauce thickens, 2 to 3 minutes.

Spoon the sauce into the squashes and cover with the parmesan and mozzarella cheeses.

Place under the oven's broiler and cook until the cheeses melt and golden brown, 2 to 3 minutes.

Remove from the oven and serve warm.

Nutrition:

Calories:865 , Total Fat:80.2g, Saturated Fat:56.8g, Total Carbs: 19g, Dietary Fiber:5g, Sugar: 5g, Protein: 28g, Sodium: 1775mg

15. Keto Pasta With Mediterranean Tofu Balls

Preparation Time: 90 minutes + overnight chilling
Servings: 4

Ingredients:

For the keto pasta:

1 cup shredded mozzarella cheese

1 egg yolk

For the sauce:
3 tbsp olive oil
2 yellow onions, chopped
6 garlic cloves, minced
2 tbsp unsweetened tomato paste

2 large tomatoes, chopped

¼ tsp saffron powder
2 cinnamon sticks
4 ½ cups vegetable broth
Salt and black pepper to taste

For the Mediterranean meatballs:

2 cups mushroom rinds
1 lb tofu

1 egg

¼ cup almond milk
6 garlic cloves, minced
Salt and black pepper to taste

½ tsp coriander powder
¼ tsp nutmeg powder
1 tbsp smoked paprika
1 ½ tsp fresh ginger paste

1 tsp cumin powder
½ tsp cayenne pepper
1 ½ tsp turmeric powder
½ tsp cloves powder

4 tbsp chopped cilantro
4 tbsp chopped scallions
4 tbsp chopped parsley
¼ cup almond flour
¼ cup olive oil

1 cup crumbled cottage cheese for serving

Directions:

For the pasta:

Pour the cheese into a medium safe-microwave bowl and melt in the microwave for 35 minutes or until melted.

Remove the bowl and allow cooling for 1 minute only to warm the cheese but not cool completely. Mix in the egg yolk until well combined.

Lay parchment paper on a flat surface, pour the cheese mixture on top and cover with another parchment paper. Using a rolling pin, flatten the dough into 1/8-inch thickness.

Take off the parchment paper and cut the dough into spaghetti strands. Place in a bowl and refrigerate overnight.

When ready to cook, bring 2 cups of water to a boil in a medium saucepan and add the pasta.

Cook for 40 seconds to 1 minute and then drain through a colander. Run cold water over the pasta and set aside to cool.

For the Mediterranean tofu balls:

In a large pot, heat the olive oil and sauté the onions until softened, 3 minutes. Stir in the garlic and cook until fragrant, 30 seconds.

Stir in the tomato paste, tomatoes, saffron, and cinnamon sticks; cook for 2 minutes and then mix in the vegetable broth, salt, and black pepper. Simmer for 20 to 25 minutes while you make the tofu balls.

In a large bowl, mix the mushroom rinds, tofu, egg, almond milk, garlic, salt, black pepper, coriander, nutmeg powder, paprika, ginger paste, cumin powder, cayenne pepper, turmeric powder, cloves powder, cilantro, parsley, 3 tablespoons of scallions, and almond flour. Form 1-inch meatballs from the mixture.

Heat the olive oil in a large skillet and fry the tofu balls in batches until brown on all sides, 10 minutes.

Put the tofu balls into the sauce, coat well with the sauce and continue cooking over low heat for 5 to 10 minutes.

Divide the pasta onto serving plates and spoon the tofu balls with sauce on top.

Garnish with the cottage cheese, remaining scallions and serve warm.

Nutrition:

Calories: 232, Total Fat:14.3g, Saturated Fat:5.4g, Total Carbs: 12g, Dietary Fiber:g4, Sugar:4 g, Protein:20 g, Sodium: 719mg

16. Seitan-Asparagus Shirataki Mix

Preparation Time: 40 minutes
Servings: 4

Ingredients:

For the angel hair shirataki:

2 (8 oz) packs angel hair shirataki

For the seitan-asparagus base:

1 lb seitan

3 tbsp olive oil

1 lb fresh asparagus, cut into 1-inch pieces

2 large shallots, finely chopped

3 garlic cloves, minced

Salt and black pepper to taste

1 cup finely grated parmesan cheese for topping

Directions:

For the angel hair shirataki:

Bring 2 cups of water to a boil in a medium pot over medium heat.

Strain the shirataki pasta through a colander and rinse very well under hot running water.

Drain properly and transfer the shirataki pasta into the boiling water. Cook for 3 minutes and strain again.

Place a dry large skillet over medium heat and stir-fry the shirataki pasta until visibly dry, 1 to 2 minutes. Take off the heat and set aside.

For the seitan -asparagus base:

Heat a large non-stick skillet over medium heat and add the seitan. Cook while breaking the lumps that form until brown, 10 minutes. Use a slotted spoon to transfer the seitan to a plate and discard the drippings.

Heat the olive oil in the skillet and sauté the asparagus until tender, 5 to 7 minutes. Stir in the shallots and garlic and cook until fragrant, 2 minutes. Season with salt and black pepper.

Stir in the seitan, shirataki and toss until well combined. Adjust the taste with salt and black pepper as desired.

Dish the food onto serving plates and garnish generously with the parmesan cheese.

Serve warm.

Nutrition:

Calories:413 , Total Fat:30.6g, Saturated Fat:12.3g, Total Carbs: 8g, Dietary Fiber:2g, Sugar: 4g, Protein:5 g, Sodium:37 mg

17. Garlic-Butter Tempeh With Shirataki Fettucine

Preparation Time: 30 minutes

Servings: 4

Ingredients:

For the shirataki fettuccine:

2 (8 oz) packs shirataki fettuccine

For the garlic-butter steak bites:

4 tbsp butter

1 lb thick-cut tempeh, cut into 1-inch cubes

Salt and black pepper to taste

4 garlic cloves, mined

2 tbsp chopped fresh parsley

1 cup freshly grated parmesan cheese

Directions:

For the shirataki fettuccine:

Boil 2 cups of water in a medium pot over medium heat.

Strain the shirataki pasta through a colander and rinse very well under hot running water.

Allow proper draining and pour the shirataki pasta into the boiling water. Cook for 3 minutes and strain again.

Place a dry skillet over medium heat and stir-fry the shirataki pasta until visibly dry, and makes a squeaky sound when stirred, 1 to 2 minutes. Take off the heat and set aside.

For the garlic-butter mushroom bites:

 Melt the butter in a large skillet, season the mushroom with salt, black pepper and cook in the butter until brown, and cooked through, 10 minutes.

Stir in the garlic and cook until fragrant, 1 minute.

Mix in the parsley and shirataki pasta; toss well and season with salt and black pepper.

Dish the food, top with the parmesan cheese and serve immediately.

Nutrition:

Calories:399 , Total Fat: 34.2g, Saturated Fat: 18.6g, Total Carbs: 10 g, Dietary Fiber:0g, Sugar: 2g, Protein:17 g, Sodium: 283mg

18. Eggplant Ragu

Preparation Time: 20 minutes
Servings: 4

Ingredients

2 tbsp butter

1 lb eggplant

Salt and black pepper to taste

1/4 cup sugar-free tomato sauce

4 tbsp chopped fresh parsley + extra for garnishing

4 large green bell peppers, Blade A, noodles trimmed

4 large red bell peppers, Blade A, noodles trimmed

1 small red onion, Blade A, noodles trimmed

1 cup grated parmesan cheese

Directions:

Heat half of the butter in a medium skillet and cook the eggplant until brown, 5 minutes. Season with salt and black pepper.

Stir in the tomato sauce, parsley, and cook for 10 minutes or until the sauce reduces by a quarter.

Stir in the bell pepper and onion noodles; cook for 1 minute and turn the heat off.

Adjust the taste with salt, black pepper, and dish the food onto serving plates.

Garnish with the parmesan cheese and more parsley; serve warm.

Nutrition:

Calories: 163, Total Fat: 9.8g, Saturated Fat:5.6 g, Total Carbs: 7 g, Dietary Fiber:2g, Sugar:4g, Protein: 13g, Sodium: 417mg

19. Thai Tofu Shirataki Stir-Fry

Preparation Time: 35 minutes

Servings: 4

Ingredients:

For the angel hair shirataki:

2 (8 oz) packs angel hair shirataki

For the teriyaki tofu base:

2 tbsp olive oil, divided

1 ¼ lb tofu, cut into bite-size pieces

Salt and black pepper to taste

1 white onion, thinly sliced

1 red bell pepper, deseeded and sliced

1 cup sliced cremini mushrooms

4 garlic cloves, minced

1 ½ cups fresh Thai basil leaves

2 tbsp toasted sesame seeds

1 tbsp chopped peanuts

1 tbsp chopped fresh scallions

For the sauce:

3 tbsp coconut aminos

2 tbsp Himalayan salt

1 tbsp hot sauce

Directions:

For the angel hair shirataki:

Boil 2 cups of water in a medium pot over medium heat.

Strain the shirataki pasta through a colander and rinse very well under hot running water.

Allow proper draining and pour the shirataki pasta into the boiling water. Cook for 3 minutes and strain again.

Place a dry skillet over medium heat and stir-fry the shirataki pasta until visibly dry, and makes a squeaky sound when stirred, 1 to 2 minutes. Take off the heat and set aside.

For the teriyaki tofu base:

Heat the olive oil in a large skillet, season the tofu with salt, black pepper, and sear in the oil on both sides until brown, 5 minutes. Transfer to a plate and set aside.

Add the onion, bell pepper, and mushrooms to the skillet; cook until softened, 5 minutes. Stir in the garlic and cook until fragrant, 1 minute.

Return the tofu to the skillet and add the pasta.

Quickly, combine the sauce's Ingredients in a small bowl: coconut aminos, Himalayan salt, and hot sauce. Pour the mixture over the tofu mix. Top with the Thai basil and toss well to coat. Cook for 1 to 2 minutes or until warmed through.

Dish the food onto serving plates and garnish with the sesame seeds, peanuts, and scallions.

Nutrition:

Calories: 598, Total Fat: 56g, Saturated Fat:18.8g, Total Carbs: 12 g, Dietary Fiber3:g, Sugar:5 g, Protein: 15g, Sodium:762 mg

20. Classic Tempeh Lasagna

Preparation Time: 70 minutes

Servings: 4

Ingredients:

For the lasagna noodles:

4 oz dairy- free cream cheese, room temperature

1 ½ cup grated mozzarella cheese

1 tsp dried Italian seasoning

2 large eggs, cracked into a bowl

For the lasagna filling:

1 lb tempeh

1 medium white onion, chopped

1 tsp Italian seasoning

Salt and black pepper to taste

1 cup sugar-free marinara sauce

6 tbsp vegan ricotta cheese

½ cup grated mozzarella cheese

½ cup grated parmesan cheese

Directions:

For the lasagna noodles:

Preheat the oven to 350 F and line a 9 x 13 –inch baking sheet with parchment paper.

In a food processor or blender, add the dairy- free cream cheese, mozzarella cheese, Italian seasoning, and eggs. Blend until well mixed.

Pour the cheese mixture on the baking sheet and spread across the pan.

Bake in the middle layer of the oven until set and firm to touch, 20 minutes.

Remove the cheese pasta and set aside to cool while you make the lasagna sauce.

For the lasagna sauce:

In a large skillet, combine the tempeh, onion and cook until brown, 5 minutes. Season with the Italian seasoning, salt, and black pepper. Cook further for 1 minute and mix in the marinara sauce. Simmer for 3 minutes. Turn the heat off.

Evenly cut the lasagna pasta into thirds making sure it fits into your baking sheet.

Spread a layer of the tempeh mixture in the baking sheet and make a first single layer on the tempeh mixture.

Spread a third of the remaining tempeh mixture on the pasta, top with a third each of the vegan ricotta cheese, mozzarella cheese, and parmesan cheese. Repeat the layering two more times using the remaining Ingredients in the same quantities.

Bake in the oven until the cheese melts and is bubbly with the sauce, 20 minutes.

Remove the lasagna, allow cooling for 2 minutes and dish onto serving plates. Serve warm

Nutrition:

Calories:435 , Total Fat:38.3g, Saturated Fat:1.2g, Total Carbs: 4 g, Dietary Fiber:1g, Sugar: 2g, Protein21: g, Sodium: 388mg

21. Creamy Sun-Dried & Parsnip Noodles

Preparation Time: 35 minutes
Servings: 4

Ingredients:

3 tbsp butter

1 lb tofu, cut into strips

Salt and black pepper to taste

4 large parsnips, peeled and Blade C noodles trimmed

1 cup sun dried tomatoes in oil, chopped

4 garlic cloves, minced

1 ¼ cup coconut cream

1 cup shaved parmesan cheese

¼ tsp dried basil

¼ tsp red chili flakes

2 tbsp chopped fresh parsley for garnishing

Directions:

Melt 1 tablespoon of butter in a large skillet, season the tofu with salt, black pepper and cook in the butter until brown, and cooked within, 8 to 10 minutes.

In another medium skillet, melt the remaining butter and sauté the parsnips until softened, 5 to 7 minutes. Set aside.

Stir in the sun-dried tomatoes and garlic into the tofu, cook until fragrant, 1 minute.

Reduce the heat to low and stir in the coconut cream and parmesan cheese. Simmer until the cheese melts. Season with the salt, basil, and red chili flakes.

Fold in the parsnips until well coated and cook for 2 more minutes.

Dish the food into serving plates, garnish with the parsley and serve warm.

Nutrition:

Calories:224 , Total Fat: 20.4g, Saturated Fat:12.2 g, Total Carbs: 1 g, Dietary Fiber:0g, Sugar: 1g, Protein: 9g, Sodium:556 mg

22. Keto Vegan Bacon Carbonara

Preparation Time: 30 minutes

Servings: 4

Ingredients:

For the keto pasta:

1 cup shredded mozzarella cheese

1 large egg yolk

For the carbonara:

4 vegan bacon slices, chopped

1¼ cups coconut whipping cream

¼ cup mayonnaise

Salt and black pepper to taste

4 egg yolks

1 cup grated parmesan cheese + more for garnishing

Directions:

For the pasta:

Pour the cheese into a medium safe-microwave bowl and melt in the microwave for 35 minutes or until melted.

Take out the bowl and allow cooling for 1 minute only to warm the cheese but not cool completely. Mix in the egg yolk until well combined.

Lay a parchment paper on a flat surface, pour the cheese mixture on top and cover with another parchment paper. Using a rolling pin, flatten the dough into 1/8-inch thickness.

Take off the parchment paper and cut the dough into thin spaghetti strands. Place in a bowl and refrigerate overnight.

When ready to cook, bring 2 cups of water to a boil in medium saucepan and add the pasta.

Cook for 40 seconds to 1 minute and then drain through a colander. Run cold water over the pasta and set aside to cool.

For the carbonara:

Add the vegan bacon to a medium skillet and cook over medium heat until crispy, 5 minutes. Set aside.

Pour the coconut whipping cream into a large pot and allow simmering for 3 to 5 minutes.

Whisk in the mayonnaise and season with the salt and black pepper. Cook for 1 minute and spoon 2 tablespoons of the mixture into a medium bowl. Allow cooling and mix in the egg yolks.

Pour the mixture into the pot and mix quickly until well combined. Stir in the parmesan cheese to melt and fold in the pasta.

Spoon the mixture into serving bowls and garnish with more parmesan cheese. Cook for 1 minute to warm the pasta.

Serve immediately.

Nutrition:

Calories:456 , Total Fat: 38.2g, Saturated Fat:14.7g, Total Carbs:13 g, Dietary Fiber:3g, Sugar: 8g, Protein:16g, Sodium:604 mg

23. Seitan Lo Mein

Preparation Time: 25 minutes
Servings: 4

Ingredients:

For the keto pasta:

1 cup shredded mozzarella cheese

1 egg yolk

For the seitan and vegetables:

1 tbsp sesame oil

3 seitan, cut into ¼-inch strips

Salt and black pepper to taste

1 red bell pepper, deseeded and thinly sliced

1 yellow bell pepper, deseeded and thinly sliced

1 cup green beans, trimmed and halved

1 garlic clove, minced

1-inch ginger knob, peeled and grated

4 green onions, chopped

1 tsp toasted sesame seeds to garnish

For the sauce:

3 tbsp coconut aminos

2 tsp sesame oil

2 tsp sugar-free maple syrup

1 tsp fresh ginger paste

Directions:

For the pasta:

Pour the cheese into a medium safe-microwave bowl and melt in the microwave for 35 minutes or until melted.

Take out the bowl and allow cooling for 1 minute only to warm the cheese but not cool completely. Mix in the egg yolk until well-combined.

Lay a parchment paper on a flat surface, pour the cheese mixture on top and cover with another parchment paper. Using a rolling pin, flatten the dough into 1/8-inch thickness.

Take off the parchment paper and cut the dough into thin spaghetti strands. Place in a bowl and refrigerate overnight.

When ready to cook, bring 2 cups of water to a boil in medium saucepan and add the pasta. Cook for 40 seconds to 1 minute and then drain through a colander. Run cold water over the pasta and set aside to cool.

For the seitan and vegetables:

Heat the sesame oil in a large skillet, season the seitan with salt, black pepper, and sear in the oil on both sides until brown, 5 minutes. Transfer to a plate and set aside.

Mix in the bell peppers, green beans and cook until sweaty, 3 minutes. Stir in the garlic, ginger, green onions and cook until fragrant, 1 minute.

Add the seitan and pasta to the skillet and toss well.

In a small bowl, toss the sauce's Ingredients: the coconut aminos, sesame oil, maple syrup, and ginger paste.

Pour the mixture over the seitan mixture and toss well; cook for 1 minute.

Dish the food onto serving plates and garnish with the sesame seeds. Serve warm.

Nutrition:
Calories:273, Total Fat:20g, Saturated Fat:11.6g, Total Carbs:6g, Dietary Fiber:1g, Sugar:4g, Protein:17g, Sodium:931mg

24. Pasta & Cheese Mushroom

Preparation Time: 1 hour 45 minutes

Servings: 4

Ingredients:

For the keto macaroni:

1 cup shredded mozzarella cheese

1 egg yolk

For the pulled mushroom mac and cheese:

2 tbsp olive oil

1 lb mushroom

Salt and black pepper to taste

1 tsp dried thyme

1 cup vegetable broth

2 tbsp butter

2 medium shallots, minced

2 garlic cloves, minced

1 cup water

1 cup grated cheddar cheese

4 oz dairy- free cream cheese, room temperature

1 cup coconut cream

½ tsp white pepper

½ tsp nutmeg powder

2 tbsp chopped parsley

Directions:

For the keto macaroni:

Pour the cheese into a medium safe-microwave bowl and melt in the microwave for 35 minutes or until melted.

Take out the bowl and allow cooling for 1 minute only to warm the cheese but not cool completely. Mix in the egg yolk until well-combined.

Lay a parchment paper on a flat surface, pour the cheese mixture on top and cover with another parchment paper. Using a rolling pin, flatten the dough into 1/8-inch thickness.

Take off the parchment paper and cut the dough into small cubes of the size of macaroni. Place in a bowl and refrigerate overnight.

When ready to cook, bring 2 cups of water to a boil in medium saucepan and add the keto macaroni. Cook for 40 seconds to 1 minute and then drain through a colander. Run cold water over the pasta and set aside to cool.

For the mushroom mac and cheese:

Heat the olive oil in a large pot, season the mushroom with salt, black pepper, thyme, and sear in the oil on both sides until brown. Pour on the vegetable broth, cover, and cook over low heat for 15 minutes or until softened. When ready, remove the mushroom onto a plate and set aside.

Preheat the oven to 380 F.

Melt the butter in a large skillet and sauté the shallots until softened. Stir in the garlic and cook until fragrant, 30 seconds.

Pour in the water to deglaze the pot and then stir in half of the cheddar cheese and dairy- free cream cheese until melted, 4 minutes. Mix in the coconut cream and season with salt, black pepper, white pepper, and nutmeg powder.

Add the pasta, mushroom, and half of the parsley to the mixture; combine well.

Pour the mixture into a baking dish and cover the top with the remaining cheddar cheese. Bake in the oven until the cheese melts and the food bubbly, 15 to 20 minutes.

Remove from the oven, allow cooling for 2 minutes and garnish with the parsley.

Serve warm.

Nutrition:
Calories:647, Total Fat:56.5g, Saturated Fat:32g, Total Carbs:6g, Dietary Fiber:1g, Sugar:2g, Protein:30g, Sodium:609mg

25. Pesto Parmesan Tempeh With Green Pasta

Preparation Time: 1 hour 27 minutes
Servings: 4

Ingredients:

4 tempeh

Salt and black pepper to taste

½ cup basil pesto, olive oil-based

1 cup grated parmesan cheese

1 tbsp butter

4 large turnips, Blade C, noodle trimmed

Directions:

Preheat the oven to 350 F.

Season the tempeh with salt, black pepper and place on a baking sheet. Divide the pesto on top and spread well on the tempeh.

Place the sheet in the oven and bake for 45 minutes to 1 hour or until cooked through.

When ready, pull out the baking sheet and divide half of the parmesan cheese on top of the tempeh. Cook further for 10 minutes or until the cheese melts. Remove the tempeh and set aside for serving.

Melt the butter in a medium skillet and sauté the turnips until tender, 5 to 7 minutes. Stir in the remaining parmesan cheese and divide between serving plates.

Top with the tempeh and serve warm.

Nutrition:
Calories:442, Total Fat:29.4g, Saturated Fat:11.3g, Total Carbs:8g, Dietary Fiber:1g, Sugar:1g, Protein:39g, Sodium:814mg

26. Creamy Tofu With Green Beans And Keto Fettuccine

Preparation Time: 40 minutes

Servings: 4

Ingredients:

For the keto fettuccine:

1 cup shredded mozzarella cheese

1 egg yolk

For the creamy tofu and green beans:

1 tbsp olive oil

4 tofu, cut into thin strips

Salt and black pepper to taste

½ cup green beans, chopped

1 lemon, zested and juiced

¼ cup vegetable broth

1 cup plain yogurt

6 basil leaves, chopped

1 cup shaved parmesan cheese for topping

Directions:

For the keto fettucine:

Pour the cheese into a medium safe-microwave bowl and melt in the microwave for 35 minutes or until melted.

Take out the bowl and allow cooling for 1 minute only to warm the cheese but not cool completely. Mix in the egg yolk until well-combined.

Lay a parchment paper on a flat surface, pour the cheese mixture on top and cover with another parchment paper. Using a rolling pin, flatten the dough into 1/8-inch thickness.

Take off the parchment paper and cut the dough into thick fettuccine strands. Place in a bowl and refrigerate overnight.

When ready to cook, bring 2 cups of water to a boil in medium saucepan and add the keto fettuccine. Cook for 40 seconds to 1 minute and then drain through a colander. Run cold water over the pasta and set aside to cool.

For the creamy tofu and green beans:

Heat the olive oil in a large skillet, season the tofu with salt, black pepper, and cook in the oil until brown on the outside and slightly cooked through, 10 minutes.

Mix in the green beans and cook until softened, 5 minutes.

Stir in the lemon zest, lemon juice, and vegetable broth. Cook for 5 more minutes or until the liquid reduces by a quarter.

Add the plain yogurt and mix well. Pour in the keto fettuccine and basil, fold in well and cook for 1 minute. Adjust the taste with salt and black pepper as desired.

Dish the food onto serving plates, top with the parmesan cheese and serve warm.

Nutrition:
Calories:721, Total Fat:76.8g, Saturated Fat:21.2g, Total Carbs:2g, Dietary Fiber:0g, Sugar:0g, Protein:9g, Sodium:309mg

27. Delicious Sambal Seitan Noodles

Preparation Time: 60 minutes

Servings: 4

Ingredients:

For the shirataki noodles:

2 (8 oz) packs Miracle noodles, garlic and herb

Salt to season

For the sambal seitan:

1 tbsp olive oil

1 lb seitan

4 garlic cloves, minced

1-inch ginger, peeled and grated

1 tsp liquid erythritol

1 tbsp sugar-free tomato paste

2 fresh basil leaves + extra for garnishing

2 tbsp sambal oelek

2 tbsp plain vinegar

1 cup water

2 tbsp coconut aminos

Salt to taste

1 tbsp unsalted butter

Directions:

For the shirataki noodles:

Bring 2 cups of water to a boil in a medium pot over medium heat.

Strain the Miracle noodles through a colander and rinse very well under hot running water.

Allow proper draining and pour the noodles into the boiling water. Cook for 3 minutes and strain again.

Place a dry skillet over medium heat and stir-fry the shirataki noodles until visibly dry, 1 to 2 minutes. Season with salt, plate and set aside.

For the seitan sambal:

Heat the olive oil in a large pot and cook in the seitan until brown, 5 minutes.

Stir in the garlic, ginger, liquid erythritol and cook for 1 minute.

Add the tomato paste, cook for 2 minutes and mix in the basil, sambal oelek, vinegar, water, coconut aminos, and salt. Cover the pot and continue cooking over low heat for 30 minutes.

Uncover, add the shirataki noodles, butter and mix well into the sauce.

Dish the food, garnish with some basil leaves and serve warm.

Nutrition:
Calories:538, Total Fat:41.1g, Saturated Fat:16.2g, Total Carbs:20g, Dietary Fiber:14g, Sugar:5g, Protein:29g, Sodium:640mg

28. Tofu Avocado Keto Noodles

Preparation Time: 15 minutes
Servings: 4

Ingredients:

2 tbsp butter

1 lb tofu

Salt and black pepper to taste

8 large red and yellow bell peppers, Blade A, noodles trimmed

1 tsp garlic powder

2 medium avocados, pitted, peeled and mashed

2 tbsp chopped pecans for topping

Directions:

Melt the butter in a large skillet and cook the tofu until brown, 5 minutes. Season with salt and black pepper.

Stir in the bell peppers, garlic powder and cook until the peppers are slightly tender, 2 minutes.

Mix in the mashed avocados, adjust the taste with salt and black pepper and cook for 1 minute.

Dish the food onto serving plates, garnish with the pecans and serve warm.

Nutrition:
Calories:209, Total Fat:15.2g, Saturated Fat:7.3g, Total Carbs:8g, Dietary Fiber:1g, Sugar:2g, Protein:13g, Sodium:468mg

29. Lemongrass Tempeh With Spaghetti Squash

Preparation Time: 1 hour + 45 minutes marinating time
Servings: 4

Ingredients:

For the lemongrass tempeh:

2 tbsp minced lemongrass

2 tbsp fresh ginger paste

2 tbsp sugar-free maple syrup

2 tbsp coconut aminos

1 tbsp Himalayan salt

4 tempeh

2 tbsp avocado oil

For the squash noodles:

3 lb spaghetti squashes, halved and deseeded

1 tbsp olive oil

Salt and black pepper to taste

For the steamed spinach:

1 tbsp avocado oil

1 tsp fresh ginger paste

1 lb baby spinach

For the peanut-coconut sauce:

½ cup coconut milk

¼ cup organic almond butter

Directions:

For the lemongrass tempeh:

In a medium bowl, mix the lemongrass, ginger paste, maple syrup, coconut aminos, and Himalayan salt. Place the tempeh in the liquid and coat well. Allow marinating for 45 minutes.

After, heat the avocado oil in a large skillet, remove the tempeh from the marinade and sear in the oil on both sides until golden brown and cooked through, 10 to 15 minutes. Transfer to a plate and cover with foil.

For the spaghetti squash:

Preheat the oven to 380 F.

Place the spaghetti squashes on a baking sheet, brush with the olive oil and season with salt and black pepper. Bake in the oven for 20 to 25 minutes or until tender.

When ready, remove the squash and shred with two forks into spaghetti-like strands. Keep warm in the oven.

For the spinach:

In another skillet, heat the avocado oil and sauté the ginger until fragrant. Add the spinach and cook to wilt while stirring to be coated well in the ginger, 2 minutes. Turn the heat off.

For the almond-coconut sauce:

In a medium bowl, quickly whisk the coconut milk with the almond butter until well combined.

To serve:

Unwrap and divide the tempeh into four bowls, add the spaghetti squash to the side, then the spinach and drizzle the almond sauce on top.

Serve immediately.

Nutrition:
Calories:457, Total Fat:37g, Saturated Fat:8.1g, Total Carbs:17g, Dietary Fiber:5g, Sugar:4g, Protein:22g, Sodium:656mg

30. Chinese Seitan And Celeriac Noodles

Preparation Time: 1 hour 18 minutes

Servings: 4

Ingredients:

3 tbsp sugar-free maple syrup

3 tbsp coconut aminos

1 tbsp fresh ginger paste

¼ tsp Chinese five spice powder

Salt and black pepper to taste

1 lb seitan, cut into 1-inch cubes

2 tbsp butter

4 medium large celeriac, peeled and Blade B noodle trimmed

1 tbsp sesame oil

4 heads baby bok choy, leaves separated

2 green onions, chopped for garnishing

2 tbsp sesame seeds for garnishing

Directions:

Preheat the oven to 400 F and line a baking sheet with foil.

In a large bowl, mix the maple syrup, coconut aminos, ginger paste, Chinese five-spice powder, salt, and black pepper. Spoon 3 tablespoons of the mixture into a small bowl and reserve for topping. Mix the seitan cubes into the remaining marinade and set aside to marinate for 25 minutes.

Meanwhile, melt the butter in a medium skillet and sauté the celeriac until softened, 5 to 7 minutes or until tender. Turn the heat off and set aside.

When the marinating is over, remove the seitan from the marinade onto the baking sheet and cook in the oven for 40 minutes or until cooked through.

When the seitan is almost ready, heat the sesame oil in a large skillet and sauté the bok choy and zucchini pasta until slightly wilted and tender, 2 to 3 minutes.

 Transfer to serving bowls and top with the seitan when ready. Garnish with the green onions and sesame seeds.

Drizzle the reserved marinade on top and serve warm.

Nutrition:

Calories:702, Total Fat:54.9g, Saturated Fat:29.6g, Total Carbs:7g, Dietary Fiber:1g, Sugar:4g, Protein:47g, Sodium:688mg

31. Garlic Pecorino Koodles With Tofu

Preparation Time: 15 minutes
Servings: 4

Ingredients:

2 tbsp olive oil

1 cup sliced tofu

4 vegan bacon slices, chopped

4 large kohlrabi, peeled and Blade B noodles trimmed

6 garlic cloves, minced

1 cup cherry tomatoes, halved

Salt and black pepper to taste

7 fresh basil leaves

1 cup grated parmesan cheese

1 tbsp pine nuts for topping

Directions:

Heat the olive oil in a large skillet and cook the tofu and vegan bacon until brown, 5 minutes. Transfer to a plate and set aside.

Stir in the kohlrabi and cook until tender, 5 to 7 minutes. Mix the garlic into the oil and cook until fragrant, 30 seconds. Then, add the cherry tomatoes, salt, and black pepper; cook for 2 minutes.

Mix in the tofu, vegan bacon, basil, and half of the parmesan cheese. Turn the heat off.

Dish the food onto serving plates and garnish with the remaining cheese and pine nuts.

Serve warm.

Nutrition:
Calories:503, Total Fat:50g, Saturated Fat:30.9g, Total Carbs:13g, Dietary Fiber:4g, Sugar:7g, Protein:4g, Sodium:49mg

32. Creamy Tuscan Tofu Linguine

Preparation Time: 35 minutes

Servings: 4

Ingredients:

For the keto linguine:

1 cup shredded mozzarella cheese

1 egg yolk

For the creamy Tuscan tofu:

2 tbsp olive oil

4 tofu

1 medium white onion, chopped

1 cup sundried tomatoes in oil, drained and chopped

1 red bell pepper, deseeded and chopped

5 garlic cloves, minced

1 tsp dried oregano

¾ cup vegetable broth

1 ½ cup coconut cream

¾ cup grated parmesan cheese

1 cup baby kale, chopped

Salt and black pepper to taste

Directions:

For the keto linguine:

Pour the cheese into a medium safe-microwave bowl and melt in the microwave for 35 minutes or until melted.

Take out the bowl and allow cooling for 1 minute only to warm the cheese but not cool completely. Mix in the egg yolk until well-combined.

Lay a parchment paper on a flat surface, pour the cheese mixture on top and cover with another parchment paper. Using a rolling pin, flatten the dough into 1/8-inch thickness.

Take off the parchment paper and cut the dough into linguine-like strands. Place in a bowl and refrigerate overnight.

When ready to cook, bring 2 cups of water to a boil in medium saucepan and add the keto linguine. Cook for 40 seconds to 1 minute and then drain through a colander. Run cold water over the pasta and set aside to cool.

For the creamy Tuscan tofu:

Heat the olive oil in a large skillet, season the tofu with salt, black pepper, and cook in the oil until golden brown on the outside and cooked within, 7 to 8 minutes. Transfer the tofu to a plate and cut into 4 slices each. Set aside.

Add the onion, sundried tomatoes, bell pepper to the skillet and sauté until softened, 5 minutes. Mix in the garlic, oregano and cook until fragrant, 1 minute.

Deglaze the skillet with the vegetable broth and mix in the coconut cream. Simmer for 2 minutes and stir in the parmesan cheese until melted, 2 minutes.

Once the cheese melts, stir in the kale to wilt and adjust the taste with salt and black pepper.

Mix in the linguine and tofu until well coated in the sauce.

Dish the food and serve warm.

Nutrition:
Calories:127, Total Fat:12.7g, Saturated Fat:4.6g, Total Carbs:1g, Dietary Fiber:0g, Sugar:0g, Protein:3g, Sodium:57mg

33. One-Pot Spicy Cheddar Pasta

Preparation Time: 35 minutes
Servings: 4

Ingredients:

For the shirataki fettuccine:

2 (8 oz) packs shirataki fettuccine

For the spicy cheddar pasta:

4 tempeh

1 medium yellow onion, minced

3 garlic cloves, minced

1 tsp Italian seasoning

½ tsp garlic powder

¼ tsp red chili flakes

¼ tsp cayenne pepper

1 cup sugar-free marinara sauce

1 cup grated mozzarella cheese

½ cup grated cheddar cheese

Salt and black pepper to taste

2 tbsp chopped parsley

Directions:

For the shirataki fettuccine:

Boil 2 cups of water in a medium pot over medium heat.

Strain the shirataki pasta through a colander and rinse very well under hot running water.

Allow proper draining and pour the shirataki pasta into the boiling water. Cook for 3 minutes and strain again.

Place a dry skillet over medium heat and stir-fry the shirataki pasta until visibly dry, and makes a squeaky sound when stirred, 1 to 2 minutes. Take off the heat and set aside.

For the spicy cheddar pasta:

Heat the olive oil in a large pot, season the tempeh with salt, black pepper, and cook in the oil until golden brown on both sides and cooked within, 10 minutes. Transfer to a plate, cut into cubes and set aside.

Add the onion and garlic to the pan and cook until softened and fragrant, 3 minutes. Season with the Italian seasoning, garlic powder, red chili flakes, and cayenne pepper. Cook for 1 minute.

Stir in the marinara sauce, cover the pot and simmer for 5 minutes. Open the lid and adjust the taste with salt and black pepper.

Reduce the heat to low and return the tempeh to the sauce as well as the shirataki fettucine, mozzarella cheese and cheddar cheese. Stir until the cheese melts.

Dish the food onto serving plates and garnish with the parsley.

Serve warm.

Nutrition:
Calories:208, Total Fat:20g, Saturated Fat:9.1g, Total Carbs:1g, Dietary Fiber:0g, Sugar:1g, Protein:7g, Sodium:446mg

34. Mushroom Alfredo Zoodles

Preparation Time: 23 minutes
Servings: 4

Ingredients:

4 tbsp butter

4 mushrooms, cut into 1-inch cubes

Salt and black pepper to taste

4 large turnips, peeled and Blade C noodle trimmed

3 garlic cloves, minced

¾ cup coconut cream

1 cup grated parmesan cheese

2 tbsp chopped fresh parsley

Directions:

Melt 2 tablespoons of butter in a large skillet, season the mushroom with salt, black pepper, and cook in the oil until golden brown on both sides and cooked within, 10 minutes. Transfer to a plate and set aside.

Melt the remaining butter in the skillet and sauté the turnips until softened, 6 minutes.

Add the garlic to the pan and cook until fragrant, 1 minute.

Reduce the heat to low and stir in the coconut cream and parmesan cheese until melted. Season with salt, black pepper.

Stir in the mushroom and dish the food onto serving plates.

Garnish with the parsley and serve warm.

Nutrition:
Calories:127, Total Fat:12.7g, Saturated Fat:4.6g, Total Carbs:1g, Dietary Fiber:0g, Sugar:0g, Protein:3g, Sodium:57mg

35. Tomato Kale Eggplant Skillet With Keto Linguine

Preparation Time: 30 minutes

Servings: 4

Ingredients:

For the keto linguine:

1 cup shredded mozzarella cheese

1 egg yolk

For the tomato-kale eggplant:

3 tbsp olive oil

4 large eggplants, cut into 1-inch pieces

Salt and black pepper to taste

1 yellow onion, chopped

4 garlic cloves, minced

1 cup cherry tomatoes, halved

½ cup vegetable broth

2 cups baby kale, chopped

1 cup grated parmesan cheese for serving

2 tbsp pine nuts for topping

Directions:

For the keto linguine:

Pour the cheese into a medium safe-microwave bowl and melt in the microwave for 35 minutes or until melted.

Take out the bowl and allow cooling for 1 minute only to warm the cheese but not cool completely. Mix in the egg yolk until well-combined.

Lay a parchment paper on a flat surface, pour the cheese mixture on top and cover with another parchment paper. Using a rolling pin, flatten the dough into 1/8-inch thickness.

Take off the parchment paper and cut the dough into linguine strands. Place in a bowl and refrigerate overnight.

When ready to cook, bring 2 cups of water to a boil in medium saucepan and add the keto linguine. Cook for 40 seconds to 1 minute and then drain through a colander. Run cold water over the pasta and set aside to cool.

For the tomato-kale eggplant:

Heat the olive oil in a medium pot, season the eggplants with salt, black pepper, and sear in the oil until golden brown on the outside. Transfer to a plate and set aside.

Add the onion and garlic to the oil and cook until softened and fragrant, 3 minutes.

Mix in the tomatoes and vegetable broth, cover and cook over low heat until the tomatoes soften and the liquid reduces by half. Season with salt and black pepper.

Return the eggplants to the pot and stir in the kale. Allow wilting for 2 minutes.

Divide the keto linguine onto serving plates, top with the kale sauce and then the parmesan cheese.

Garnish with the pine nuts and serve warm.

Nutrition:
Calories:442, Total Fat:39.9g, Saturated Fat:18.5g, Total Carbs:15g, Dietary Fiber:1g, Sugar:2g, Protein:7g, Sodium:274mg

36. Mustard Tofu Shirataki

Preparation Time: 40 minutes

Servings: 4

Ingredients:

For the shirataki angel hair:

2 (8 oz) packs angel hair shirataki

For the mustard sauce:

1 tbsp olive oil

4 tofu, cut into strips

Salt and black pepper to taste

1 medium yellow onion, finely sliced

1 medium yellow bell pepper, deseeded and thinly sliced

1 garlic clove, minced

1 tbsp wholegrain mustard

5 tbsp coconut cream

1 cup chopped mustard greens

1 tbsp chopped parsley

Directions:

For the shirataki angel hair:

Boil 2 cups of water in a medium pot over medium heat.

Strain the shirataki pasta through a colander and rinse very well under hot running water.

Allow proper draining and pour the shirataki pasta into the boiling water. Cook for 3 minutes and strain again.

Place a dry skillet over medium heat and stir-fry the shirataki pasta until visibly dry, and makes a squeaky sound when stirred, 1 to 2 minutes. Take off the heat and set aside.

For the mustard tofu sauce:

Heat the olive oil in a large skillet, season the tofu with salt, black pepper, and cook in the oil until golden brown on the outside and cooked through, 8 to 10 minutes. Transfer to a plate and set aside.

Stir in the onion, bell pepper and cook until softened, 5 minutes. Mix in the garlic and cook until fragrant, 30 seconds.

Mix in the mustard and coconut cream; simmer for 2 minutes and mix in the tofu and mustard greens. Allow wilting for 2 minutes and adjust the taste with salt and black pepper.

Stir in the shirataki pasta, allow warming for 1 minute and dish the food onto serving plates.

Garnish with the parsley and serve warm.

Nutrition:
Calories:375, Total Fat:32.1g, Saturated Fat:17.8g, Total Carbs:6g, Dietary Fiber:2g, Sugar:4g, Protein:15g, Sodium:237mg

37. Bacon Beef Pasta Time

Servings: 8
Preparation Time: 5 minutes
Cooking time: 40–45 minutes

Ingredients

1 pound extra-lean ground beef

8 slices center-cut bacon

1 large onion, chopped

2 cloves garlic, minced

3 cups mushrooms, quartered

2 (14½-ounce) cans diced tomatoes, undrained

1 (24-ounce) jar pasta sauce

1½ cups water

3 cups penne pasta

1 cup Colby & Monterey Jack cheeses, shredded

¼ cup fresh parsley, chopped

Directions

To a large skillet or saucepan, add the bacon and cook over medium-high heat until crispy. Set aside, drain on paper towel and crumble.

Clean the skillet and add the mushrooms, ground beef, onions and garlic.

Stir-cook until lightly browned.

Add half of the crumbled bacon on top; mix in the water, tomatoes, pasta and pasta sauce.

Boil the mixture.

Cover and allow the mixture to simmer for 18–20 minutes over medium-low heat, stirring periodically, until the pasta is cooked to your satisfaction.

Take the pasta mixture off the heat.

Top with the remaining bacon and cheese.

Set aside until the cheese melts and top with some parsley. Serve warm.

Nutrition:

Calories 400, fat 11 g, carbs 49 g, protein 25 g, sodium 570 mg

38. Italian Orecchiette Sausage Feast

Servings: 2
Preparation Time: 15 minutes
Cooking time: 25 minutes

Ingredients

½ pound spicy Italian sausages, casings removed

3½ cups low-sodium chicken broth

1¼ cups orecchiette pasta

2 tablespoons olive oil

½ onion, diced

Salt to taste

½ cup arugula, roughly chopped

¼ cup Parmesan cheese, finely grated

Directions

Add the oil to a large skillet or saucepan and heat it over medium heat.

Add the onions and a pinch of salt and sauté while stirring until softened, about 5–7 minutes.

Add the sausage; stir-cook until browned, about 5–7 minutes, and break into small pieces.

Pour in 1½ cups of the chicken broth and allow the mixture to boil.

Mix in the pasta and remaining broth.

Cook the mixture, stirring periodically, until the pasta is cooked to your satisfaction and the liquid evaporates, about 14–15 minutes.

Add the arugula; stir and cook until it wilts.

Take the pasta mixture off the heat.

Top with the cheese and serve warm.

Nutrition:

Calories 662, fat 39 g, carbs 46 g, protein 31 g, sodium 1360 mg

39. Tortellini Sausage Spinach

Servings: 4
Preparation Time: 5 minutes
Cooking time: 15 minutes

Ingredients

½ pound smoked sausage, sliced into ½-inch rounds

2 cloves garlic, minced

1 tablespoon olive oil

½ cup half-and-half

10 ounces tortellini pasta

2 (14-ounce) cans fire-roasted diced tomatoes

2–3 cups baby spinach, roughly chopped

Salt and ground black pepper to taste

Directions

Add the oil to a large skillet and heat it over medium heat.

Add the sausage and stir-cook until lightly browned.

Add the garlic and sauté while stirring until softened, about 30 seconds.

Mix in the cream and tomatoes; simmer the mixture.

Mix in the pasta. Cook the mixture, stirring periodically, until the pasta is cooked to your satisfaction, about 8–10 minutes.

Season with salt and pepper to taste. Mix in the chopped spinach; cook until wilted.

Serve warm.

Nutrition:

Calories 728, fat 28 g, carbs 62 g, protein 28 g, sodium 1147 mg

40. Broccoli Pork Orecchiette

Servings: 4
Preparation Time: 5 minutes
Cooking time: 20–25 minutes

Ingredients

1 tablespoon olive oil

1 pound broccoli rabe leaves, stemmed and roughly chopped

1 pound spicy Italian-style pork (or chicken) sausage

2 cloves garlic, minced

Pinch red pepper flakes (optional)

3 cups whole wheat or regular orecchiette

1 quart low-sodium chicken broth

Kosher salt and freshly ground black pepper to taste

2 tablespoons fresh lemon juice

1 teaspoon lemon zest

½ cup Parmesan cheese, grated

Breadcrumbs to taste

Directions

Add the oil to a large skillet and heat it over medium-high heat.

Add the sausage and stir-cook until no longer pink, about 3–4 minutes. Break it into small pieces and set aside in a container.

In the skillet, sauté the broccoli for about 2 minutes until it turns soft and wilted. Add to the sausage container.

Reserve 1 tablespoon of fat in the skillet and discard the rest.

Add the garlic and pepper flakes and sauté while stirring until fragrant, about 30 seconds.

Mix in the broth and pasta.

Cook the mixture, stirring periodically, until the pasta is cooked to your satisfaction, about 8–9 minutes.

Add the broccoli and sausage; stir and cook for 3–4 more minutes.

Take the pasta mixture off the heat, season to taste with black pepper and salt, and mix in the zest and lemon juice.

Mix in the cheese. Top with the breadcrumbs and serve warm.

Nutrition:

Calories 746, fat 36 g, carbs 45 g, protein 42 g, sodium 1863 mg

41. Spinach Lamb Whole Wheat Pasta

Servings: 5
Preparation Time: 5 minutes
Cooking time: 25–30 minutes

Ingredients

6 cups chopped spinach

½ pound whole-wheat elbow noodles

1 pound ground lamb

1 (14-ounce) can unsalted diced tomatoes

1 medium onion, chopped

4 cloves garlic, thinly sliced

2 tablespoons tahini paste

1 teaspoon dried oregano

1 teaspoon ground cumin

¾ teaspoon salt

1 quart water

2 tablespoons crumbled feta cheese

Directions

To a large cooking pot, add the lamb, pasta, tahini, spinach, onion, tomatoes, garlic, cumin, oregano and salt.

Stir in the water and heat over medium-high heat.

Allow the pasta mixture to boil gradually.

Cook the mixture, stirring periodically, until the pasta is cooked to your satisfaction, about 10–12 minutes.

Take the pasta mixture off the heat.

Top with the feta cheese and serve warm.

Nutrition:

Calories 400, fat 16 g, carbs 42 g, protein 24 g, sodium 444 mg

42. Bacon Whole Wheat Pasta

Servings: 4
Preparation Time: 5 minutes
Cooking time: 15 minutes

Ingredients

3 strips bacon, preferably thick cut

½ pound whole wheat pasta

2 cups water or broth

2 cloves garlic, minced

⅓ cup crumbled blue cheese

¼ cup chopped sun dried tomatoes

2 tablespoons milk

Walnuts and parsley (optional, for garnishing)

Directions

To a large skillet or saucepan, add the bacon and cook over medium-high heat until crispy. Set aside half the cooked bacon, drain on paper towels and crumble.

Break the remaining bacon into chunks; stir in the pasta, water, garlic or broth, and tomatoes.

Cover and boil the mixture.

Allow the mixture to simmer for 7–8 minutes, until the pasta is cooked to your satisfaction.

Take the pasta mixture off the heat and mix in the milk and cheese. Combine until the cheese melts.

Top with the reserved bacon, walnuts and parsley and serve warm.

Nutrition:

Calories 504, fat 9 g, carbs 64 g, protein 22 g, sodium 274 mg

43. Tomato Lamb Gemelli

Servings: 6
Preparation Time: 5 minutes
Cooking time: 35–40 minutes

Ingredients

1 tablespoon olive oil

1 medium onion, chopped

2 cloves garlic, minced

15 ounces ground lamb

3 tablespoons tomato paste

1 teaspoon salt

¼ teaspoon red chili flakes

1 tablespoon fresh rosemary, chopped

3 cups tomatoes, diced

2 cups unsalted beef or chicken broth

3½ cups gemelli or other small pasta

Directions

Add the oil to a large cooking pot and heat it over medium heat.

Add the onions and garlic and sauté while stirring until softened, about 3–4 minutes.

Increase the heat and mix in the lamb. Break it into small pieces. Stir-cook until lightly browned, about 5–7 minutes.

Mix in the tomato paste, rosemary, salt and pepper flakes; stir-cook for 2 minutes. Stir in the broth and tomatoes; allow the mixture to boil gradually.

Turn down heat to low. Allow the mixture to simmer for 14–15 minutes.

Mix in the pasta and boil the mixture.

Allow the mixture to simmer for 10 minutes, until the pasta is cooked to your satisfaction.

Serve warm.

Nutrition:

Calories 383, fat 14 g, carbs 42 g, protein 21 g, sodium 486 mg

44. Sausage Fennel Pasta Meal

Servings: 4–6
Preparation Time: 5 minutes
Cooking time: 15–20 minutes

Ingredients

1 (14½-ounce) can fire-roasted diced tomatoes

½ fennel bulb, thinly sliced

1 cup fresh basil leaves, torn

¾ pound linguine

¾ pound smoked Andouille sausage, cut into ½-inch pieces

1 tablespoon kosher salt

½ teaspoon freshly ground pepper

2 tablespoons olive oil

4½ cups water

Directions

Add the oil to a large skillet or saucepan along with the tomatoes, pasta, basil, fennel, sausage, water, black pepper and salt.

Stir and heat over medium-high heat.

Allow the pasta mixture to boil gradually.

Cook the mixture, stirring periodically, until the pasta is cooked to your satisfaction, about 8–9 minutes.

Top with some basil and serve warm.

Nutrition:

Calories 328, fat 18 g, carbs 23 g, protein 10 g, sodium 985 mg

45. Wine Beef Pasta Meal

Servings: 6
Preparation Time: 5 minutes
Cooking time: 30 minutes

Ingredients

1 pound ground beef

1 stalk celery, chopped

3 cloves garlic, minced

1 large onion, chopped

1 medium carrot, chopped

1 teaspoon dried oregano or 1 tablespoon fresh oregano, chopped

1 cup low-sodium beef broth

½ cup red wine

1 cup tomatoes, crushed

¼ teaspoon ground black pepper (or to taste)

½ teaspoon salt (or to taste)

3 cups low-sodium vegetable broth

1 pound fettuccine or other pasta

2 tablespoons parsley, chopped (for garnish)

Parmesan cheese, grated (for serving)

Directions

Add the beef to a large Dutch oven or deep saucepan and stir-cook over medium-high heat until lightly browned, about 5 minutes. Break into small pieces.

Add the onions, celery and carrot and sauté while stirring until softened, about 4–5 minutes.

Mix in the wine, garlic, oregano, tomatoes and beef broth. Season with salt and pepper.

Mix in the vegetable broth and pasta. Cook the mixture, stirring periodically, until the pasta is cooked to your satisfaction, about 18–20 minutes.

Take the pasta mixture off the heat.

Top with the Parmesan cheese and parsley; serve warm.

Nutrition:

Calories 480, fat 11 g, carbs 63 g, protein 27 g, sodium 871 mg

46. Worcestershire Beef Macaroni

Servings: 6
Preparation Time: 20 minutes
Cooking time: 65 minutes

Ingredients

2 large yellow onions, chopped

6 cloves garlic, chopped

2 pounds lean ground beef

2 (15-ounce) cans tomato sauce

2 (14½-ounce) cans diced tomatoes

3 cups water

3 tablespoons Worcestershire sauce

½ cup sofrito sauce

2 tablespoons Italian seasoning

1 tablespoon seasoned salt (or to taste)

2½ cups elbow macaroni

3 bay leaves

Directions

Add the beef to a large cooking pot or Dutch oven and stir-cook over medium-high heat until lightly browned, about 8–10 minutes.

Remove the grease. Add the onions and garlic and sauté while stirring until softened, about 9–10 minutes.

Mix in the tomatoes, tomato sauce, water, Worcestershire sauce, sofrito, Italian seasoning, bay leaves and salt.

Boil the mixture and then turn down heat to low.

Cover and allow the mixture to simmer for 18–20 minutes.

Mix in the macaroni, cover and allow the mixture to simmer for 25 minutes, until the pasta is cooked to your satisfaction.

Remove the bay leaves and serve warm.

Nutrition:

Calories 442, fat 18 g, carbs 45 g, protein 28 g, sodium 1271 mg

47. Cheesy Beef Pasta

Servings: 6
Preparation Time: 5 minutes
Cooking time: 30 minutes

Ingredients

1 pound ground beef

1 cup onion, diced

1 tablespoon garlic, minced

1 teaspoon salt

½ teaspoon ground black pepper

2 tablespoons Worcestershire sauce

2 tablespoons ketchup

1 quart beef broth

1 pound fusilli pasta

3 cups cheddar cheese, shredded

½ cup milk

Sliced green onions to serve

Directions

To a large cooking pot, add the garlic, ground beef, onions, salt, pepper, ketchup and Worcestershire sauce. Stir-cook over medium-high heat until lightly browned, about 6–7 minutes. Break the beef into small pieces.

Stir in the water and broth; simmer the mixture.

Mix in the pasta. Cook the mixture, stirring periodically, until the pasta is cooked to your satisfaction, about 18–20 minutes.

Mix in the milk and cheese. Stir until the cheese melts completely

Serve warm with green onions on top.

Nutrition:

Calories 702, fat 31 g, carbs 56 g, protein 42 g, sodium 1458 mg

48. Beef Bucatini Pasta

Servings: 4
Preparation Time: 5 minutes
Cooking time: 25–30 minutes

Ingredients

2 tablespoons extra-virgin olive oil

3 cloves garlic, chopped

1 medium onion, finely chopped

3 sprigs fresh thyme

2 medium carrots, finely chopped

2 stalks celery, finely chopped

1 pound 80–85% lean ground beef chuck

2 tablespoons tomato paste

3 cups water

¼ teaspoon freshly ground black pepper

2½ teaspoons kosher salt (divided) + more for serving

1 (28-ounce) can diced tomatoes

¾ pound bucatini, broken in half

¼ cup Parmesan cheese, grated + more for serving

¼ cup fresh parsley, chopped + more for serving

Directions

Add the oil to a large skillet or saucepan and heat it over medium-high heat.

Add the onions, celery, carrot, garlic, thyme and ½ teaspoon of salt and sauté while stirring until softened, about 5–7 minutes.

Stir in the tomato paste and cook for 1 minute.

Add the beef, ¼ teaspoon of pepper and 1 teaspoon of salt. Cook while stirring until lightly browned, about 4–5 minutes. Break the beef into small pieces.

Add the bucatini, water, tomatoes and 1 teaspoon of salt. Combine the mixture.

Allow the pasta mixture to boil gradually. Cook the mixture, stirring periodically, until the pasta is cooked to your satisfaction, about 10–12 minutes.

Take the pasta mixture off the heat, remove the thyme sprigs, and mix in the parsley and Parmesan cheese. Season to taste with salt.

Top with additional parsley and Parmesan cheese and serve warm.

Nutrition:

Calories 758, fat 27 g, carbs 52 g, protein 39 g, sodium 426 mg

49. Cinnamon Lamb Orzo

Servings: 4
Preparation Time: 5 minutes
Cooking time: 40–45 minutes

Ingredients

1 red onion, diced

2 tablespoons olive oil

1 clove garlic, crushed

2 teaspoons dried oregano

2 teaspoons ground cinnamon

14 ounces lean lamb, minced

1½ cups lamb stock

7 ounces orzo

14 ounces tomatoes, chopped

1 chunk feta cheese

2 sprigs fresh parsley, chopped

Directions

Add the oil to a large skillet or saucepan and heat it over medium-high heat.

Add the onions and sauté while stirring until softened.

Add the garlic, lamb, cinnamon and oregano and sauté while stirring until softened and lightly browned.

Add the stock and chopped tomatoes; simmer the mixture for 30 minutes.

Mix in the pasta and cook the mixture, stirring periodically, until the pasta is cooked to your satisfaction, about 8 minutes.

Take the pasta mixture off the heat.

Top with the parsley and feta cheese and serve warm.

Nutrition:

Calories 296, fat 13 g, carbs 21 g, protein 22 g, sodium 86 mg

50. Corn Beef & Macaroni

Servings: 6
Preparation Time: 10 minutes
Cooking time: 20 minutes

Ingredients

¼ cup onion, chopped

1 pound ground beef

2 teaspoons chili powder

2¼ cups hot water

17 ounces whole kernel corn

1 (7¼-ounce) package macaroni and cheese mix

1 (14½-ounce) can diced tomatoes

Directions

To a large cooking pot, add the onion and beef and stir-cook over medium-high heat until lightly browned, about 5–7 minutes. Break the beef into small pieces.

Remove the grease and season the cooked mix with the chili powder.

Add the water and allow the mixture to boil gradually.

Add the pasta, corn and tomatoes.

Simmer the mixture, stirring periodically, until the pasta is cooked to your satisfaction, about 8–10 minutes.

Serve warm.

Nutrition:

Calories 350, fat 11.5 g, carbs 41 g, protein 21 g, sodium 445 mg

51. Beef Bean Chili Pasta

Servings: 4
Preparation Time: 10 minutes
Cooking time: 20 minutes

Ingredients

½ pound ground beef

1 quart chicken broth

1 tablespoon olive oil

2 cloves garlic, minced

1 onion, diced

1 (14½-ounce) can diced tomatoes

¾ cup canned kidney beans, drained and rinsed

¾ cup canned white kidney beans, drained and rinsed

2 teaspoons chili powder

1½ teaspoons cumin

Kosher salt and freshly ground black pepper to taste

¾ cup cheddar cheese, shredded

10 ounces elbow pasta

2 tablespoons fresh parsley leaves, chopped

Directions

Add the oil to a large Dutch oven or skillet and heat it over medium-high heat.

Add the onions, beef and garlic and sauté while stirring until softened and evenly browned, about 4–5 minutes.

Remove the excess fat.

Mix in the beans, broth, tomatoes, chili powder and cumin; season with black pepper and salt to taste.

Simmer the mixture and stir in the pasta. Allow the pasta mixture to boil gradually.

Cover and turn down heat to low.

Simmer the mixture, stirring periodically, until the pasta is cooked to your satisfaction, about 13–15 minutes.

Take the pasta mixture off the heat and mix in the cheese until melts.

Top with the parsley and serve warm.

Nutrition:

Calories 647, fat 19 g, carbs 84 g, protein 37 g, sodium 671 mg

52. Veggie Beef Ramen

Servings: 5–6
Preparation Time: 10 minutes
Cooking time: 15 minutes

Ingredients

1 package mushroom flavor ramen noodles

2 packages chicken flavor ramen noodles

1 pound ground beef

¼ teaspoon garlic powder

¼ teaspoon dried thyme

2 cups frozen mixed vegetables

2 cups water

Directions

Remove the flavor packets from the ramen packs and set aside. Break the noodles into small chunks.

Add the beef to a large skillet and stir-cook over medium-high heat until no longer pink.

Remove the fat and add the mushroom flavor packet to the skillet; combine and cook for 2 minutes. Set aside the cooked beef mix.

Add the water to the skillet and boil it. Add the noodles, thyme, garlic power and veggies along with the chicken flavor packets.

Combine and boil the mixture.

Turn down heat to low. Cover and allow the mixture to simmer for a few minutes until the pasta is cooked to your satisfaction.

Add the beef mix and stir the mixture. Serve warm.

Nutrition:

Calories 410, fat 14 g, carbs 45 g, protein 23 g, sodium 483 mg

53. Beef Mushroom Ravioli

Servings: 4
Preparation Time: 10 minutes
Cooking time: 25–30 minutes

Ingredients

½ pound mushrooms, sliced

1 teaspoon vegetable oil

1 pound lean ground beef

1 small onion, diced

2 cloves garlic, minced

1 cup water

2 (26-ounce) jars tomato-basil or other tomato-based pasta sauce

1 tablespoon Italian seasoning

½ teaspoon salt

¼ teaspoon pepper

1 cup mozzarella cheese, shredded

1 (20-ounce) package four-cheese or regular ravioli

Directions

To a large cooking pot or Dutch oven, add the beef and stir-cook over medium-high heat until no longer pink.

Remove the excess fat and set aside the cooked beef.

Add the onions and mushrooms and sauté while stirring until softened and tender, about 7–8 minutes.

Add the garlic and sauté while stirring until softened, about 1 minute.

Mix in the water, cooked beef and other ingredients except for the pasta and cheese.

Boil the mixture and add the pasta.

Turn down heat to low. Cover and allow the mixture to simmer for 8–10 minutes, until the pasta is cooked to your satisfaction.

Take the pasta mixture off the heat and mix in the cheese. Serve warm.

Nutrition:

Calories 589, fat 26 g, carbs 37 g, protein 35 g, sodium 1658 mg

54. Spinach Chicken Casserole

Serving: 6
Preparation Time: 20 Minutes
Cooking Time: 20 Minutes

Ingredients

2 cups uncooked penne pasta

3/4 pound boneless skinless chicken breasts, cubed

1 small onion, chopped

1/2 cup chopped green pepper

1 jar (26 ounces) spaghetti sauce

1 package (16 ounces) frozen leaf spinach, thawed and squeezed dry

1 jar (6 ounces) sliced mushrooms, drained

1 can (2-1/4 ounces) sliced ripe olives, drained

2 cups shredded part-skim mozzarella cheese, divided

Direction

Cook pasta according to package directions. Meanwhile, in a large nonstick saucepan coated with cooking spray, sauté chicken until no longer pink; set aside.

In the same pan, sauté onion and green pepper until crisp-tender. Add the spaghetti sauce, spinach, mushrooms and olives. Bring to a boil. Reduce heat; simmer, uncovered, for 5 minutes. Drain pasta; add chicken and pasta to the pan. Sprinkle with 1 cup cheese and toss to coat.

Transfer to a 13x9-in. baking dish coated with cooking spray; sprinkle with remaining cheese. Cover and bake at 350 degrees for 20-25 minutes or until cheese is melted.

Nutrition:

Calories: 492 calories

Total Fat: 20g

Cholesterol: 78mg

Sodium: 1323mg

Total Carbohydrate: 38g

Protein: 39g

Fiber: 5g

55. Spinach Lasagna Rollups

Serving: 6
Preparation Time: 30 Minutes
Cooking Time: 25 Minutes

Ingredients

12 uncooked lasagna noodles

2 large eggs, lightly beaten

1 package (10 ounces) frozen chopped spinach, thawed and squeezed dry

2-1/2 cups whole-milk ricotta cheese

2-1/2 cups shredded part-skim mozzarella cheese

1/2 cup grated Parmesan cheese

1/4 teaspoon salt

1/4 teaspoon pepper

1/4 teaspoon ground nutmeg

1 jar (24 ounces) meatless pasta sauce

Direction

Preheat oven to 375 degrees. Cook and drain noodles according to package directions. Meanwhile, mix eggs, spinach, cheeses and seasonings.

Pour 1 cup pasta sauce into an ungreased 13x9-in. baking dish. Spread 1/3 cup cheese mixture over each noodle; roll up and place over sauce, seam side down. Top with remaining sauce. Bake, covered, 20 minutes. Uncover; bake until heated through, 5-10 minutes.

Nutrition:

Calories: 569 calories

Total Fat: 22g

Cholesterol: 145mg

Sodium: 1165mg

Total Carbohydrate: 57g

Protein: 38g

Fiber: 5g

56. Spinach Manicotti

Serving: 7
Preparation Time: 20 Minutes
Cooking Time: 01 h 10 Minutes

Ingredients

1 carton (15 ounces) fat-free ricotta cheese

2 cups shredded part-skim mozzarella cheese, divided

1 package (10 ounces) frozen chopped spinach, thawed and squeezed dry

1/2 cup reduced-fat sour cream

1/4 cup dry bread crumbs

1 tablespoon Italian seasoning

1 teaspoon garlic powder

1 teaspoon onion powder

2 cups tomato juice

1 cup chunky salsa

1 can (15 ounces) crushed tomatoes

14 uncooked manicotti shells

Direction

In a large bowl, combine the ricotta, 1-1/2 cups mozzarella cheese, spinach, sour cream, bread crumbs, Italian seasoning, garlic powder and onion powder.

Combine the tomato juice, salsa and crushed tomatoes; spread 1 cup sauce in an ungreased 13x9-in. baking dish. Stuff uncooked manicotti with spinach mixture; arrange over sauce. Pour remaining sauce over manicotti.

Cover and bake at 350 degrees for 55 minutes. Uncover; sprinkle with remaining mozzarella cheese. Bake 15 minutes longer or until noodles are tender.

Nutrition:

Calories: 345 calories

Total Fat: 8g

Cholesterol: 34mg

Sodium: 782mg

Total Carbohydrate: 45g

Protein: 22g

Fiber: 4g

57. Spinach Noodle Casserole

Serving: 12-14
Preparation Time: 15 Minutes
Cooking Time: 40 Minutes

Ingredients

4 cups uncooked egg noodles

1/4 cup butter, cubed

1/4 cup all-purpose flour

1 teaspoon salt

1/8 teaspoon pepper

2 cups 2% milk

2 packages (10 ounces each) frozen chopped spinach, thawed and drained

2 cups shredded Swiss cheese

2 cups shredded part-skim mozzarella cheese

1/4 cup grated Parmesan cheese

Paprika, optional

Direction

Cook noodles according to package directions; drain and rinse in cold water. Meanwhile, in a large saucepan, melt butter over medium heat. Stir in the flour, salt and pepper until smooth. Gradually add milk. Bring to a boil; cook and stir for 2 minutes or until thickened.

Arrange half of the noodles in an ungreased 11x7-in. baking dish; layer half of the spinach and half of the Swiss cheese. Spread with half of the white sauce. Repeat layers. Layer with mozzarella and Parmesan cheeses. Sprinkle with paprika if desired.

Cover and bake at 350 degrees for 20 minutes. Uncover; bake 20 minutes longer. Let stand for 15 minutes before cutting.

Nutrition:

Calories: 210 calories

Total Fat: 12g

Cholesterol: 48mg

Sodium: 378mg

Total Carbohydrate: 13g

Protein: 12g

Fiber: 1g

58. Spinach Salad With Tortellini Roasted Onions

Serving: 6
Preparation Time: 20 Minutes
Cooking Time: 20 Minutes

Ingredients

2 cups chopped sweet onion (about 1 large)

1 tablespoon canola oil

1 package (9 ounces) refrigerated cheese tortellini

1/2 to 2/3 cup Italian salad dressing, divided

1 tablespoon red wine vinegar

10 ounces fresh baby spinach (about 12 cups)

2 cups cubed cooked chicken breast (about 10 ounces)

1 can (12 ounces) marinated quartered artichoke hearts, drained

1 can (2-1/4 ounces) sliced ripe olives, drained

1/2 cup julienned roasted sweet red peppers

1/2 cup shaved Parmesan cheese

Direction

Preheat oven to 425 degrees. Toss onion with oil; spread into a foil-lined 15x10x1-in. baking pan. Roast until softened and lightly browned, 20-25 minutes, stirring occasionally.

Cook tortellini according to package directions. Drain and rinse gently with cold water; drain well.

Place 1/2 cup salad dressing, vinegar and roasted onion in a blender. Cover; process until blended, thinning with additional dressing if desired.

To serve, place spinach, chicken, artichoke hearts, olives, peppers and tortellini in a large bowl; toss with onion mixture. Top with cheese.

Nutrition:

Calories: 448 calories

Total Fat: 22g

Cholesterol: 59mg

Sodium: 887mg

Total Carbohydrate: 33g

Protein: 24g

Fiber: 3g

59. Spinach Turkey Noodle Bake

Serving: 6
Preparation Time: 20 Minutes
Cooking Time: 45 Minutes

Ingredients

2-1/2 cups uncooked yolk-free noodles

2 cups diced cooked turkey breast

1 can (10-3/4 ounces) reduced-fat reduced-sodium condensed cream of chicken soup, undiluted

1/4 teaspoon garlic salt

1/8 teaspoon dried rosemary, crushed

Dash pepper

1 package (10 ounces) frozen chopped spinach, thawed and squeezed dry

1 cup (8 ounces) fat-free cottage cheese

3/4 cup shredded part-skim mozzarella cheese, divided

1/8 teaspoon paprika

Direction

Cook noodles according to package directions; drain. Meanwhile, in a large bowl, combine the turkey, soup, garlic salt, rosemary and pepper. In another bowl, combine the spinach, cottage cheese and 1/2 cup mozzarella cheese.

In a 2-qt. baking dish coated with cooking spray, layer half of the noodles, turkey mixture and cottage cheese mixture. Repeat layers.

Cover and bake 350 degrees for 35 minutes. Uncover; sprinkle with remaining mozzarella cheese. Bake 10-15 minutes longer or until edges are lightly browned; sprinkle with paprika. Let stand for 5 minutes before serving.

Nutrition:

Calories: 242 calories

Total Fat: 4g

Cholesterol: 53mg

Sodium: 568mg

Total Carbohydrate: 21g

Protein: 26g

Fiber: 3g

60. Spinach Vegetable Lasagna

Serving: 12
Preparation Time: 30 Minutes
Cooking Time: 25 Minutes

Ingredients

3 tablespoons butter

1/2 cup all-purpose flour

2-3/4 cups fat-free milk, divided

1-1/2 cups plus 2 tablespoons grated Parmesan cheese, divided

3 tablespoons Dijon mustard

1/2 teaspoon salt, divided

1/4 teaspoon hot pepper sauce

1/2 pound sliced fresh mushrooms

2 medium onions, chopped

2 cups chopped carrots

4 garlic cloves, minced

1 tablespoon olive oil

1 pound fresh spinach, chopped

9 lasagna noodles, cooked, rinsed and drained

Direction

In a large saucepan, melt butter. Stir in flour until smooth. Add 2-1/2 cups milk. Bring to a boil; cook and stir for 1-2 minutes or until thickened. Remove from the heat. Stir in 1-1/2 cups Parmesan cheese, mustard, 1/4 teaspoon salt and hot pepper sauce; set aside.

In a large nonstick skillet, sauté the mushrooms, onions, carrots and garlic in oil until tender. Stir in spinach and remaining salt. Cook and stir for 2 minutes or until spinach is wilted; drain.

Remove from the heat; stir in 1-1/2 cups cheese sauce. Combine the remaining cheese sauce and milk. Spread half of the cheese sauce in a 13-in. x 9-in. baking dish coated with cooking spray. Top with three noodles and half the vegetable mixture; repeat. Top with remaining noodles and cheese sauce. Sprinkle with remaining cheese. Bake, uncovered, at 375 degrees for

25-30 minutes or until heated through. Let stand for 10 minutes before cutting.

Nutrition:

Calories: 222 calories

Total Fat: 8g

Cholesterol: 17mg

Sodium: 496mg

Total Carbohydrate: 27g

Protein: 12g

Fiber: 3g

61. Spinachbasil Lasagna

Serving: 9
Preparation Time: 20 Minutes
Cooking Time: 45 Minutes

Ingredients
1 large egg, lightly beaten
2 cups reduced-fat ricotta cheese
4 ounces crumbled feta cheese
1/4 cup grated Parmesan cheese
1/4 cup chopped fresh basil
2 garlic cloves, minced
1/4 teaspoon pepper
1 jar (24 ounces) pasta sauce
9 no-cook lasagna noodles
3 cups fresh baby spinach
2 cups shredded part-skim mozzarella cheese
Direction
Preheat oven to 350 degrees. Mix first seven ingredients.

Spread 1/2 cup pasta sauce into a greased 13x9-in. baking dish. Layer with three lasagna noodles, 3/4 cup ricotta mixture, 1 cup spinach, 1/2 cup mozzarella cheese and 2/3 cup sauce. Repeat layers twice. Sprinkle with remaining mozzarella cheese.

Bake, covered, 35 minutes. Uncover; bake until heated through and cheese is melted, 10-15 minutes. Let stand 5 minutes before serving. Freeze option: Cover and freeze unbaked lasagna. To use, partially thaw in refrigerator overnight. Remove from refrigerator 30 minutes before baking. Preheat oven to 350 degrees. Bake lasagna as directed, increasing time as necessary to heat through and for a thermometer inserted in center to read 165 degrees.

Nutrition:

Calories: 292 calories

Total Fat: 12g

Cholesterol: 59mg

Sodium: 677mg

Total Carbohydrate: 27g

Protein: 18g

Fiber: 3g

62. Spinachbeef Spaghetti Pie

Serving: 8
Preparation Time: 20 Minutes
Cooking Time: 20 Minutes

Ingredients

6 ounces uncooked angel hair pasta

2 large eggs, lightly beaten

1/3 cup grated Parmesan cheese

1 pound ground beef

1/2 cup chopped onion

1/4 cup chopped green pepper

1 jar (14 ounces) meatless pasta sauce

1 teaspoon Creole seasoning

3/4 teaspoon garlic powder

1/2 teaspoon dried basil

1/2 teaspoon dried oregano

1 package (8 ounces) cream cheese, softened

1 package (10 ounces) frozen chopped spinach, thawed and squeezed dry

1/2 cup shredded part-skim mozzarella cheese

Direction

Cook pasta according to package directions; drain. Add eggs and Parmesan cheese. Press onto the bottom and up the sides of a greased 9-in. deep-dish pie plate. Bake at 350 degrees for 10 minutes.

Meanwhile, in a skillet, cook the beef, onion and green pepper over medium heat until meat is no longer pink; drain. Stir in pasta sauce and seasonings. Bring to a boil. Reduce heat; cover and simmer for 10 minutes.

Between two pieces of waxed paper, roll out cream cheese into a 7-in. circle. Place in crust. Top with spinach and meat sauce. Sprinkle with mozzarella cheese. Bake at 350 degrees for 20-30 minutes or until set.

Nutrition:

Calories: 377 calories

Total Fat: 21g

Cholesterol: 130mg

Sodium: 544mg

Total Carbohydrate: 24g

Protein: 22g

Fiber: 3g

63. Spinachpork Stuffed Shells

Serving: 2
Preparation Time: 25 Minutes
Cooking Time: 25 Minutes

Ingredients

6 uncooked jumbo pasta shells

1/4 pound ground pork

4 cups water

3 cups torn fresh spinach

1 egg, lightly beaten

3 tablespoons shredded Parmesan cheese, divided

2 tablespoons heavy whipping cream

1 garlic clove, minced

1/4 teaspoon salt

1/8 teaspoon ground nutmeg

1/8 teaspoon pepper

1 cup meatless spaghetti sauce

Direction

Cook pasta shells according to package directions. Meanwhile, in a small skillet, cook pork over medium heat until no longer pink; drain and set aside. In a saucepan, bring water to a boil. Add spinach; boil for 1-2 minutes or until wilted. Drain and squeeze dry; chop the spinach.

In a bowl, combine the pork, spinach, egg, 1 tablespoon Parmesan cheese, cream, garlic, salt, nutmeg and pepper. Drain shells; stuff with the pork mixture. Spread 1/4 cup spaghetti sauce in an ungreased 1-qt. baking dish.

Place stuffed shells in dish; drizzle with remaining spaghetti sauce. Sprinkle with remaining Parmesan cheese. Cover and bake at 400 degrees for 15 minutes. Uncover; bake 10-15 minutes longer or until heated through.

Nutrition:

Calories: 379 calories

Total Fat: 15g

Cholesterol: 45mg

Sodium: 1064mg

Total Carbohydrate: 36g

Protein: 25g

Fiber: 4g

64. Spinachstuffed Chicken With Linguine

Serving: 4
Preparation Time: 20 Minutes
Cooking Time: 25 Minutes

Ingredients

3 garlic cloves, minced

1/3 cup butter, divided

1 package (6 ounces) fresh baby spinach

1/4 cup shredded Parmesan cheese

1/4 teaspoon salt

4 boneless skinless chicken breast halves (6 ounces each)

1/2 cup ricotta cheese

1 large egg, beaten

3/4 cup seasoned bread crumbs

8 ounces uncooked linguine

1/2 cup salsa

Direction

In a large skillet, sauté garlic in 1 tablespoon butter until tender. Add spinach and cook just until wilted. Remove from the heat; stir in Parmesan cheese and salt.

Flatten chicken to 1/4-in. thickness. Spread ricotta cheese and spinach mixture over the center of each chicken breast. Roll up and secure with toothpicks.

Place egg in a shallow bowl. Place bread crumbs in a separate shallow bowl. Dip chicken in egg, then coat with crumbs. In a large skillet, brown chicken in 2 tablespoons butter. Place chicken, seam side down, in a greased 11x7-in. baking dish.

Bake, uncovered, at 375 degrees for 25-30 minutes or until a thermometer reads 170 degrees.

Meanwhile, cook linguine according to package directions. Drain linguine; toss with remaining butter and salsa. Discard toothpicks from chicken. Serve with linguine.

Nutrition:

Calories: 681 calories

Total Fat: 27g

Cholesterol: 203mg

Sodium: 848mg

Total Carbohydrate: 57g

Protein: 52g

Fiber: 3g

65. Spirals And Cheese

Serving: 6
Preparation Time: 15 Minutes
Cooking Time: 20 Minutes

Ingredients

3-1/2 cups uncooked spiral pasta

4 tablespoons butter, divided

3 tablespoons all-purpose flour

3 cups 2% milk

2-1/2 cups shredded cheddar cheese, divided

3/4 cup grated Parmesan cheese, divided

1/2 teaspoon salt

1/2 teaspoon pepper

1/2 cup dry bread crumbs

Direction

Cook pasta according to package directions. Meanwhile, in a Dutch oven, melt 3 tablespoons butter. Stir in flour until smooth; gradually add milk. Bring to a boil; cook and stir for 2 minutes or until thickened. Add 2 cups cheddar cheese, 1/2 cup Parmesan cheese, salt and pepper.

Drain pasta. Add to cheese mixture; toss gently to coat. Transfer to a greased 11x7-in. baking dish. Melt remaining butter; add bread crumbs and remaining cheddar and Parmesan cheeses. Sprinkle over top. Bake, uncovered, at 400 degrees for 20-25 minutes or until golden brown.

Nutrition:

Calories: 569 calories

Total Fat: 27g

Cholesterol: 88mg

Sodium: 817mg

Total Carbohydrate: 54g

Protein: 26g

Fiber: 2g

66. Squash Pasta Bake

Serving: 2
Preparation Time: 20 Minutes
Cooking Time: 5 Minutes

Ingredients

1/2 cup chopped yellow summer squash

1/2 cup chopped zucchini

1 teaspoon olive oil

1 cup cooked small pasta shells or small tube pasta

1 cup spaghetti sauce

3 tablespoons shredded mozzarella cheese

Direction

In a skillet, sauté squash in oil for 2-3 minutes or until tender. Stir in pasta and spaghetti sauce; heat through. Transfer to a greased 3-cup baking dish. Sprinkle with cheese. Bake, uncovered, at 350 degrees for 5-10 minutes or until heated through and cheese is melted.

Nutrition:

Calories: 241 calories

Total Fat: 10g

Cholesterol: 11mg

Sodium: 661mg

Total Carbohydrate: 31g

Protein: 8g

Fiber: 4g

67. Stuffed Shells Florentine

Serving: 8-10
Preparation Time: 15 Minutes
Cooking Time: 30 Minutes

Ingredients

1 package (12 ounces) jumbo pasta shells

1 egg, lightly beaten

2 cartons (15 ounces each) ricotta cheese

1 package (10 ounces) frozen chopped spinach, thawed and squeezed dry

1/2 cup grated Parmesan cheese

1/2 teaspoon salt

1/2 teaspoon dried oregano

1/4 teaspoon pepper

1 jar (32 ounces) spaghetti sauce

Thin breadsticks, optional

Direction

Cook pasta shells according to package directions. Meanwhile, in a large bowl, combine the egg, ricotta cheese, spinach, Parmesan cheese, salt, oregano and pepper. Drain shells and rinse in cold water; stuff with spinach mixture.

Place shells in a greased 13-in. x 9-in. baking dish. Pour spaghetti sauce over shells. Cover and bake at 350 degrees for 30-40 minutes or until heated through. Serve with breadsticks if desired.

Nutrition:

Calories: 292 calories

Total Fat: 10g

Cholesterol: 44mg

Sodium: 727mg

Total Carbohydrate: 38g

Protein: 15g

Fiber: 3g

68. Stuffed Shells With Arrabbiata Sauce

Serving: 12
Preparation Time: 30 Minutes
Cooking Time: 20 Minutes

Ingredients

1 package (12 ounces) jumbo pasta shells

1 pound ground beef or turkey

1/2 pound fresh chorizo or bulk spicy pork sausage

1/2 large onion, chopped (about 1 cup)

3 garlic cloves, minced

1 package (10 ounces) frozen chopped spinach, thawed and squeezed dry

3/4 teaspoon salt, divided

1/2 teaspoon pepper, divided

1 carton (15 ounces) part-skim ricotta cheese

3/4 cup grated Parmesan cheese

2 large eggs, lightly beaten

1/4 cup chopped fresh basil

2 tablespoons chopped fresh parsley

ARRABBIATA SAUCE:

2 tablespoons olive oil

6 ounces sliced pancetta, coarsely chopped

2 teaspoons crushed red pepper flakes

2 garlic cloves, minced

2 jars (24 ounces each) marinara sauce

1-1/2 cups shredded part-skim mozzarella cheese

Direction

Preheat oven to 400 degrees. Cook pasta according to package directions for al dente. Drain and rinse in cold water.

In a large skillet, cook and crumble beef and chorizo with onion and garlic over medium heat until meat is no longer pink and vegetables are tender, 6-

8 minutes; drain. Stir in spinach, 1/2 teaspoon salt and 1/4 teaspoon pepper. Transfer to a bowl; cool.

Stir ricotta and Parmesan cheeses, eggs, basil, parsley and remaining salt and pepper into meat mixture. For sauce, in a saucepan, heat oil over medium heat. Add pancetta; cook and stir until golden brown, 6-8 minutes. Add pepper flakes and garlic; cook and stir 1 minute. Add marinara sauce; bring to a simmer.

Spread 1 cup sauce into a greased 13x9-in. baking dish. Fill pasta shells with meat mixture; place in baking dish, overlapping ends slightly. Top with remaining sauce. Sprinkle with mozzarella cheese. Bake until heated through and cheese is melted, 20-25 minutes.

Nutrition:

Calories:

Total Fat: g

Cholesterol: mg

Sodium: mg

Total Carbohydrate: g

Protein: g

Fiber: g

69. Sunday Shrimp Pasta Bake

Serving: 8
Preparation Time: 30 Minutes
Cooking Time: 25 Minutes

Ingredients

12 ounces uncooked vermicelli

1 medium green pepper, chopped

5 green onions, chopped

6 tablespoons butter, cubed

6 garlic cloves, minced

2 tablespoons all-purpose flour

2 pounds cooked medium shrimp, peeled and deveined

1 teaspoon celery salt

1/8 teaspoon pepper

1 pound process cheese (Velveeta), cubed

1 can (10 ounces) diced tomatoes and green chilies, drained

1 can (4 ounces) mushroom stems and pieces, drained

1 tablespoon grated Parmesan cheese

Direction

Preheat oven to 350 degrees. Cook vermicelli according to package directions.

Meanwhile, in a large skillet, sauté green pepper and onions in butter until tender. Add garlic; cook 1 minute longer. Gradually stir in flour until blended. Stir in shrimp, celery salt and pepper; cook, uncovered, over medium heat 5-6 minutes or until heated through.

In a microwave-safe bowl, combine process cheese, tomatoes and mushrooms. Microwave, uncovered, on high 3-4 minutes or until cheese is melted, stirring occasionally. Add to shrimp mixture. Drain vermicelli; stir into skillet. Pour into a greased 13x9-in. baking dish. Sprinkle with Parmesan cheese.

Bake, uncovered, 25-30 minutes or until heated through.

Nutrition:

Calories: 558 calories

Total Fat: 25g

Cholesterol: 281mg

Sodium: 1410mg

Total Carbohydrate: 42g

Protein: 42g

Fiber: 3g

70. Sunflower Slaw

Serving: 66(3/4 cup each).
Preparation Time: 15 Minutes
Cooking Time: 10 Minutes

Ingredients

6 packages (3 ounces each) ramen noodles

2 packages (2-1/4 ounces each) slivered almonds

1-1/3 cups sunflower kernels

1/2 cup butter, melted

3-1/2 cups canola oil

2 cups sugar

2 cups cider vinegar

1/2 cup soy sauce

2 teaspoons salt

10 pounds cabbage, shredded

Direction

Break noodles into small pieces (save seasoning packets for another use). Place the noodles, almonds and sunflower kernels in 15x10x1-in. baking pan. Drizzle with butter; toss to coat. Bake at 350 degrees for 8-10 minutes or until lightly browned, stirring several times; set aside.

Combine the oil, sugar, vinegar, soy sauce and salt; toss with cabbage. Cover and refrigerate for at least 1 hour. Stir in noodle mixture just before serving. Serve with a slotted spoon.

Nutrition:

Calories: 185 calories

Total Fat: 15g

Cholesterol: 4mg

Sodium: 231mg

Total Carbohydrate: 12g

Protein: 2g

Fiber: 2g

71. Sweet Potato Sausage Casserole

Serving: 8
Preparation Time: 20 Minutes
Cooking Time: 25 Minutes

Ingredients

8 ounces uncooked spiral pasta

8 ounces Johnsonville TM ; Fully Cooked Smoked Sausage Rope, cut into 1/4 inch slices

2 medium sweet potatoes, peeled and cut into 1/2 inch cubes

1 cup chopped green pepper

1/2 cup chopped onion

2 tablespoons olive oil

1 teaspoon minced garlic

1 can (14-1/2 ounces) diced tomatoes, undrained

1 cup heavy whipping cream

1/4 teaspoon salt

1/4 teaspoon pepper

1 cup shredded cheddar cheese

Direction

Cook pasta according to package directions. Meanwhile, in a large skillet, cook the sausage, sweet potatoes, green pepper and onion in oil over medium heat for 5 minutes or until vegetables are tender. Add garlic; cook 1 minute longer. Drain.

Add the tomatoes, cream, salt and pepper. Bring to a boil; remove from the heat. Drain pasta; stir into sausage mixture. Transfer to a greased 13x9-in. baking dish. Sprinkle with cheese.

Bake, uncovered, at 350 degrees for 25-30 minutes or until bubbly. Let stand for 5 minutes before serving.

Nutrition:

Calories:

Total Fat: g

Cholesterol: mg

Sodium: mg

Total Carbohydrate: g

Protein: g

Fiber: g

72. Swiss Cheese Lasagna

Serving: 12
Preparation Time: 60 Minutes
Cooking Time: 40 Minutes

Ingredients

1 pound ground beef

1 large onion, chopped

1 garlic clove, minced

3 cups water

1 can (12 ounces) tomato paste

2 teaspoons salt

1/2 to 1 teaspoon dried rosemary, crushed

1/4 teaspoon pepper

1 package (8 ounces) lasagna noodles

8 ounces sliced Swiss cheese

1-1/2 cups (12 ounces each) 4% cottage cheese

1/2 cup shredded part-skim mozzarella cheese

Direction

In a large skillet, cook the beef, onion and garlic over medium heat until meat is no longer pink; drain. Stir in the water, tomato paste, salt, rosemary and pepper. Bring to a boil. Reduce heat; simmer, uncovered, for 30 minutes.

Meanwhile, cook lasagna noodles according to package directions; drain. In a greased 13-in. x 9-in. baking dish, layer a third of the meat sauce, noodles and Swiss cheese. Repeat layers. Top with cottage cheese and the remaining Swiss cheese, noodles and sauce. Sprinkle with mozzarella cheese.

Cover and bake at 350 degrees for 30 minutes. Uncover; bake 10-15 minutes longer or until bubbly. Let stand for 10 minutes before serving.

Nutrition:

Calories: 275 calories

Total Fat: 11g

Cholesterol: 48mg

Sodium: 596mg

Total Carbohydrate: 23g

Protein: 20g

Fiber: 3g

73. Swiss Macaroni

Serving: 6-8
Preparation Time: 20 Minutes
Cooking Time: 30 Minutes

Ingredients

1 package (7 ounces) elbow macaroni

1 jar (2 ounces) diced pimientos, drained

2 large eggs, lightly beaten

1 cup half-and-half cream

1 small onion, chopped

2 tablespoons minced fresh parsley

1-1/2 teaspoons salt

1/8 teaspoon pepper

1 cup soft bread crumbs

1 cup shredded Swiss cheese

1/4 cup butter, melted

Direction

Cook macaroni according to package directions; drain and place in a greased 11x7-in. baking dish. Stir in the pimientos. In a large bowl, combine the eggs, cream, onion, parsley, salt and pepper.

Pour over macaroni mixture. Sprinkle with bread crumbs and cheese; drizzle with butter. Bake, uncovered, at 350 degrees for 30 minutes or until golden brown.

Nutrition:

Calories: 269 calories

Total Fat: 14g

Cholesterol: 96mg

Sodium: 600mg

Total Carbohydrate: 24g

Protein: 10g

Fiber: 1g

74. Swiss Tuna Bake

Serving: 4
Preparation Time: 10 Minutes
Cooking Time: 20 Minutes

Ingredients

4 cups cooked egg noodles

1-1/2 cups shredded Swiss cheese

1 cup mayonnaise

1 can (6 ounces) tuna, drained and flaked

1 cup seasoned bread crumbs, divided

Direction

In a large bowl, combine the noodles, cheese, mayonnaise and tuna. Sprinkle 1/2 cup bread crumbs into a greased 9-in. square baking dish. Spread noodle mixture over crumbs. Sprinkle with the remaining crumbs. Bake, uncovered, at 350 degrees for 18-22 minutes or until heated through.

Nutrition:

Calories: 856 calories

Total Fat: 59g

Cholesterol: 106mg

Sodium: 987mg

Total Carbohydrate: 48g

Protein: 32g

Fiber: 2g

75. Taco Noodle Bake

Serving: 8
Preparation Time: 20 Minutes
Cooking Time: 10 Minutes

Ingredients

2 cups uncooked wide egg noodles

2 pounds ground beef

1 can (8 ounces) tomato sauce

1/2 cup water

1 can (4 ounces) chopped green chilies

1 envelope taco seasoning

1 teaspoon onion powder

1 teaspoon chili powder

1/2 teaspoon garlic powder

1 cup shredded cheddar cheese

2 cups shredded lettuce

1 cup diced fresh tomatoes

1/3 cup sliced ripe olives, drained

1/2 cup taco sauce

1/2 cup sour cream

Direction

Preheat oven to 350 degrees. Cook noodles according to package directions.

Meanwhile, in a large skillet, cook beef over medium heat until no longer pink; drain. Stir in tomato sauce, water, green chilies, taco seasoning, onion powder, chili powder and garlic powder. Bring to a boil. Reduce heat; simmer, uncovered, 5 minutes.

Drain noodles; place in a greased 11x7-in. baking dish. Spread with beef mixture; sprinkle with cheese. Bake, uncovered, 10-15 minutes or until cheese is melted. Let stand 10 minutes.

Top with lettuce, tomatoes, olives and taco sauce. Garnish with sour cream.

Nutrition:

Calories: 402 calories

Total Fat: 23g

Cholesterol: 119mg

Sodium: 906mg

Total Carbohydrate: 17g

Protein: 30g

Fiber: 2g

76. Tangy Meatballs Over Noodles

Serving: 8(40 meatballs).
Preparation Time: 25 Minutes
Cooking Time: 50 Minutes

Ingredients

1 egg, lightly beaten

1/3 cup milk

1/4 cup seasoned bread crumbs

1 tablespoon dried minced onion

1 teaspoon salt

1-1/2 pounds ground beef

2 cans (14-3/4 ounces each) beef gravy

1/2 cup packed brown sugar

1/4 cup cider vinegar

3/4 teaspoon ground ginger

1/4 teaspoon ground cloves

1 package (12 ounces) egg noodles

Direction

In a large bowl, combine the first five ingredients. Crumble beef over mixture and mix well. Shape into 1-1/2-in. balls. Place meatballs on a greased rack in a shallow pan. Bake, uncovered, at 350 degrees for 20 minutes; drain.

With a slotted spoon, transfer meatballs into a greased 2-1/2-qt. baking dish. Combine gravy, brown sugar, vinegar, ginger and cloves; pour over meatballs. Cover and bake 30 minutes longer or until meat is no longer pink. Meanwhile, cook noodles according to package directions; drain. Serve with meatballs.

Nutrition:

Calories: 435 calories

Total Fat: 14g

Cholesterol: 127mg

Sodium: 747mg

Total Carbohydrate: 51g

Protein: 26g

Fiber: 1g

77. Tasty Chicken Noodle Casserole

Serving: 2 casseroles (8-10 each).
Preparation Time: 20 Minutes
Cooking Time: 35 Minutes

Ingredients

1 package (16 ounces) egg noodles

1 medium sweet red pepper, chopped

1 large onion, chopped

1 celery rib, chopped

1/4 cup butter, cubed

2 garlic cloves, minced

1-1/2 cups sliced fresh mushrooms

3 tablespoons all-purpose flour

3 cups chicken broth

3 cups half-and-half cream

2 packages (8 ounces each) cream cheese, cubed

12 cups cubed cooked chicken

1 to 1-1/2 teaspoons salt

TOPPING:

1 cup finely crushed cornflakes

2 tablespoons butter, melted

1 tablespoon canola oil

3 tablespoons minced fresh parsley

1/2 teaspoon paprika

Direction

Cook noodles according to package directions; drain. In a large skillet, sauté the red pepper, onion and celery in butter until tender. Add garlic; cook 1 minute longer. Add mushrooms; cook 2-3 minutes or until tender. Remove vegetables with a slotted spoon; set aside.

Add flour to the skillet; stir until blended. Gradually add broth. Bring to a boil; cook and stir for 2 minutes or until thickened. Reduce heat. Gradually stir in cream. Add the cream cheese; cook and stir until cheese is melted. Remove from the heat.

In a large bowl, combine the chicken, salt, noodles, vegetables and cheese sauce. Transfer to two ungreased shallow 3-qt. baking dishes.

Combine topping ingredients. Sprinkle over top. Cover and bake at 350 degrees for 20 minutes. Uncover; bake 15-20 minutes longer or until bubbly.

Nutrition:

Calories: 399 calories

Total Fat: 19g

Cholesterol: 136mg

Sodium: 455mg

Total Carbohydrate: 24g

Protein: 31g

Fiber: 1g

78. Tempting Turkey Casserole

Serving: 3
Preparation Time: 15 Minutes
Cooking Time: 25 Minutes

Ingredients

3 ounces uncooked spaghetti, broken into 2-inch pieces

1/2 cup process cheese sauce, warmed

1/4 cup 2% milk

1-1/2 cups frozen chopped broccoli, thawed

3/4 cup cubed cooked turkey

1/3 cup canned mushroom stems and pieces, drained

1 tablespoon pimientos, chopped

1/8 to 1/4 teaspoon onion powder

1/8 teaspoon poultry seasoning

Direction

Cook spaghetti according to package directions. Meanwhile, in a small bowl, whisk cheese sauce and milk. Add the broccoli, turkey, mushrooms, pimientos, onion powder and poultry seasoning. Drain pasta; add to broccoli mixture.

Transfer to a 1-qt. baking dish coated with cooking spray. Cover and bake at 350 degrees for 25-30 minutes or until heated through.

Nutrition:

Calories: 313 calories

Total Fat: 12g

Cholesterol: 55mg

Sodium: 838mg

Total Carbohydrate: 29g

Protein: 22g

Fiber: 3g

79. Texmex Pasta

Serving: 4
Preparation Time: 15 Minutes
Cooking Time: 15 Minutes

Ingredients

2 cups uncooked spiral pasta

1 pound ground beef

1 jar (16 ounces) salsa

1 can (10-3/4 ounces) condensed cream of chicken soup, undiluted

1 cup shredded Mexican cheese blend, divided

Direction

Preheat oven to 350 degrees. Cook pasta according to package directions.

Meanwhile, cook beef in a Dutch oven over medium heat until no longer pink; drain. Stir in the salsa, soup and 1/2 cup cheese; heat through.

Drain pasta; stir into meat mixture. Transfer to a greased 11x7-in. baking dish. Sprinkle with remaining cheese. Cover and bake 15-20 minutes or until cheese is melted.

Nutrition:

Calories: 585 calories

Total Fat: 28g

Cholesterol: 101mg

Sodium: 1241mg

Total Carbohydrate: 46g

Protein: 33g

Fiber: 3g

80. Thanksgiving Stuffed Shells

Serving: 8
Preparation Time: 25 Minutes
Cooking Time: 15 Minutes

Ingredients

24 uncooked jumbo pasta shells

1 cup shredded part-skim mozzarella cheese

1 cup cubed cooked turkey

1 cup cooked stuffing

4 green onions, chopped

1 cup mashed sweet potatoes

1/4 teaspoon chili powder, optional

1/2 cup grated Parmesan cheese

1 cup turkey gravy, warmed

Direction

Preheat oven to 350 degrees. Cook shells according to package directions for al dente.

Meanwhile, in a large bowl, mix mozzarella cheese, turkey, stuffing and green onions. In a small bowl, stir sweet potatoes and, if desired, mix in chili powder.

Drain shells; fill each with 2 tablespoons stuffing mixture and 2 teaspoons sweet potato mixture. Arrange in a greased 11x7-in. baking dish; sprinkle with Parmesan cheese. Bake, covered, 15-20 minutes or until heated through. Serve with gravy.

Nutrition:

Calories:

Total Fat: g

Cholesterol: mg

Sodium: mg

Total Carbohydrate: g

Protein: g

Fiber: g

81. Threecheese Pepper Penne

Serving: 2 casseroles (5each).
Preparation Time: 40 Minutes
Cooking Time: 30 Minutes

Ingredients

1 package (16 ounces) penne pasta

1-1/2 pounds boneless skinless chicken breasts, cut into 1/2-inch pieces

1-1/4 teaspoons salt

1/2 teaspoon pepper

3 teaspoons olive oil, divided

1 pound sliced fresh mushrooms

4 garlic cloves, minced

1/4 cup butter, cubed

1/2 cup all-purpose flour

4 cups 2% milk

2 jars (7 ounces each) roasted sweet red peppers, drained and chopped

2 cups shredded mozzarella and provolone cheese

2 cups grated Parmesan cheese, divided

Direction

Cook pasta according to package directions. Meanwhile, sprinkle chicken with salt and pepper. In a large skillet, sauté chicken in 1 teaspoon oil until no longer pink. Remove from the skillet. In the same skillet, sauté mushrooms in remaining oil until tender.

In a Dutch oven, sauté garlic in butter for 1 minute. Stir in flour until blended; gradually add milk. Bring to a boil; cook and stir for 1-2 minutes or until thickened. Stir in the red peppers, mozzarella and provolone cheese, 1/2 cup Parmesan cheese, mushrooms and chicken.

Drain pasta; stir into sauce. Divide between two greased 8-in. square baking dishes. Sprinkle each with remaining Parmesan cheese.

Cover and freeze one casserole for up to 3 months. Cover and bake the remaining casserole at 350 degrees for 30-35 minutes or until bubbly.

To use frozen casserole: Thaw in the refrigerator overnight. Remove from the refrigerator 30 minutes before baking. Cover and bake at 350 degrees for 60-70 minutes or until bubbly, stirring once.

Nutrition:

Calories: 534 calories

Total Fat: 21g

Cholesterol: 87mg

Sodium: 1002mg

Total Carbohydrate: 47g

Protein: 37g

Fiber: 2g

82. Threecheese Pasta Shells

Serving: 8
Preparation Time: 15 Minutes
Cooking Time: 40 Minutes

Ingredients

1 jar (16 ounces) salsa

1 can (8 ounces) no-salt-added tomato sauce

1/2 cup shredded carrots

1/2 cup shredded zucchini

1/2 cup sliced fresh mushrooms

1/4 cup chopped green onions

1 garlic clove, minced

1 teaspoon canola oil

1 carton (15 ounces) reduced-fat ricotta cheese

1/4 cup grated Parmesan cheese

1/4 cup shredded part-skim mozzarella cheese

1/4 cup egg substitute

2 teaspoons dried basil

16 jumbo pasta shells, cooked and drained

Direction

In a bowl, combine the salsa and tomato sauce; spread half in an 11x7-in. baking dish coated with cooking spray.

In a skillet, sauté the carrot, zucchini, mushrooms, onions and garlic in oil until crisp-tender. Remove from the heat. Stir in the cheeses, egg substitute and basil. Stuff into pasta shells; place in prepared baking dish. Top with the remaining salsa mixture. Cover and bake at 350 degrees for 40-45 minutes or until heated through.

Nutrition:

Calories: 203 calories

Total Fat: 7g

Cholesterol: 21mg

Sodium: 416mg

Total Carbohydrate: 23g

Protein: 12g

Fiber: 2g

83. Threecheese Sausage Lasagna

Serving: 12
Preparation Time: 30 Minutes
Cooking Time: 30 Minutes

Ingredients

1-1/2 pounds Johnsonville TM ; Ground Mild Italian sausage

6 tablespoons butter

6 tablespoons all-purpose flour

1 teaspoon salt

1 teaspoon pepper

3 cups 2% milk

9 lasagna noodles, cooked and drained

6 slices part-skim mozzarella cheese, cut in half

6 slices provolone cheese, cut in half

1/3 cup grated Romano cheese

Direction

In a large skillet, cook sausage over medium heat until no longer pink; drain and set aside.

In a small saucepan, melt butter. Stir in the flour, salt and pepper until smooth; gradually stir in milk. Bring to a boil over medium heat; cook and stir for 2 minutes or until thickened. Remove from the heat.

In a greased 13-in. x 9-in. baking dish, layer with a fourth of the white sauce, three noodles, half of the sausage and four pieces each of mozzarella and provolone cheeses. Repeat layers once. Spoon half of the remaining sauce over the top. Layer with remaining noodles, sauce, mozzarella and provolone cheeses; sprinkle with Romano cheese.

Bake, uncovered, at 350 degrees for 30-35 minutes or until heated through. Let stand for 15 minutes before cutting.

Nutrition:

Calories: 350 calories

Total Fat: 21g

Cholesterol: 64mg

Sodium: 756mg

Total Carbohydrate: 21g

Protein: 18g

Fiber: 1g

84. Threecheese Shells

Serving: 9
Preparation Time: 20 Minutes
Cooking Time: 30 Minutes

Ingredients

1 package (12 ounces) jumbo pasta shells

3 cups ricotta cheese

3 cups shredded part-skim mozzarella cheese

1/2 cup grated Parmesan cheese

1/2 cup chopped green pepper

1/2 cup chopped fresh mushrooms

2 tablespoons dried basil

2 large eggs, lightly beaten

2 garlic cloves, minced

1/2 teaspoon seasoned salt

1/4 teaspoon pepper

2 jars (one 28 ounces, one 14 ounces) spaghetti sauce, divided

Direction

Cook pasta shells according to package directions. Drain and rinse in cold water. In a large bowl, combine the next 10 ingredients. Divide the small jar of spaghetti sauce between two ungreased 13x9-in. baking dishes.

Stuff shells with the cheese mixture and place in a single layer over sauce. Pour the remaining spaghetti sauce over shells.

Cover and bake at 350 degrees for 20 minutes. Uncover; bake 10 minutes longer or until heated through.

Nutrition:

Calories: 512 calories

Total Fat: 24g

Cholesterol: 116mg

Sodium: 1084mg

Total Carbohydrate: 47g

Protein: 29g

Fiber: 4g

85. Tofu Manicotti

Serving: 5
Preparation Time: 25 Minutes
Cooking Time: 50 Minutes

Ingredients

2 cups meatless spaghetti sauce

1 can (14-1/2 ounces) diced tomatoes, undrained

1/3 cup finely shredded zucchini

1/4 cup finely shredded carrot

1/2 teaspoon Italian seasoning

1 package (12.3 ounces) silken firm tofu

1 cup 1% cottage cheese

1 cup shredded part-skim mozzarella cheese

1 tablespoon grated Parmesan cheese

10 uncooked manicotti shells

Direction

Combine the spaghetti sauce, tomatoes, zucchini, carrot and Italian seasoning; spread 3/4 cup into a 13x9-in. baking dish coated with cooking spray.

Combine the tofu and cheeses; stuff into uncooked manicotti shells. Place over spaghetti sauce; top with remaining sauce.

Cover and bake at 375 degrees for 50-55 minutes or until noodles are tender. Let stand for 5 minutes before serving.

Nutrition:

Calories: 319 calories

Total Fat: 7g

Cholesterol: 16mg

Sodium: 885mg

Total Carbohydrate: 42g

Protein: 23g

Fiber: 4g

86. Tofu Spinach Lasagna

Serving: 12
Preparation Time: 45 Minutes
Cooking Time: 30 Minutes

Ingredients

9 lasagna noodles

1 medium onion, chopped

3 garlic cloves, minced

1 tablespoon olive oil

2 cups sliced fresh mushrooms

1 package (14 ounces) firm tofu

1 carton (15 ounces) part-skim ricotta cheese

1/2 cup minced fresh parsley

1 teaspoon salt, divided

2 packages (10 ounces each) frozen chopped spinach, thawed and squeezed dry

1-3/4 cups marinara or meatless spaghetti sauce

1 cup shredded part-skim mozzarella cheese

1/3 cup shredded Parmesan cheese

Direction

Cook noodles according to package directions. Meanwhile, in a large nonstick skillet, sauté onion and garlic in oil for 1 minute. Add mushrooms; sauté until tender. Set aside.

Drain tofu, reserving 2 tablespoons liquid. Place tofu and reserved liquid in a food processor; cover and process until blended. Add ricotta cheese; cover and process for 1-2 minutes or until smooth. Transfer to a large bowl; stir in the parsley, 1/2 teaspoon salt and mushroom mixture. Combine spinach and remaining salt; set aside.

Drain noodles. Spread half of the marinara sauce into a 13x9-in. baking dish coated with cooking spray. Layer with three noodles, half of the tofu mixture and half of the spinach mixture. Repeat layers of noodles, tofu and spinach. Top with remaining noodles and marinara sauce. Sprinkle with cheeses.

Bake, uncovered, at 350 degrees for 30-35 minutes or until heated through and cheese is melted. Let stand for 10 minutes before cutting.

, ,

Nutrition:

Calories: 227 calories

Total Fat: 8g

Cholesterol: 18mg

Sodium: 429mg

Total Carbohydrate: 25g

Protein: 15g

Fiber: 3g

87. Tofustuffed Pasta Shells

Serving: 5
Preparation Time: 25 Minutes
Cooking Time: 35 Minutes

Ingredients

15 uncooked jumbo pasta shells

1-1/2 cups silken firm tofu

3 tablespoons grated Romano cheese, divided

2 garlic cloves, peeled

1 package (10 ounces) frozen chopped spinach, thawed and squeezed dry

1 can (14-1/2 ounces) Italian diced tomatoes, drained

1 can (8 ounces) tomato sauce

1/4 cup dry red wine or vegetable broth

1/2 cup shredded part-skim mozzarella cheese

Direction

Cook pasta shells according to package directions. Meanwhile, in a blender, combine the tofu, 2 tablespoons Romano cheese and garlic; cover and process until smooth. (Add 1 tablespoon water if mixture is too thick.) Add spinach; process until blended. Drain shells; stuff with tofu mixture.

In a small bowl, combine the tomatoes, tomato sauce and wine. Spread about 1/2 cup sauce in an 11x7-in. baking dish coated with cooking spray. Arrange stuffed shells over sauce. Top with remaining sauce.

Cover and bake at 350 degrees for 25 minutes. Uncover; sprinkle with mozzarella and remaining Romano cheese. Bake 8-10 minutes longer or until shells are heated through and cheese is melted.

Nutrition:

Calories: 262 calories

Total Fat: 5g

Cholesterol: 10mg

Sodium: 754mg

Total Carbohydrate: 39g

Protein: 14g

Fiber: 4g

88. Tomato N Cheese Pasta

Serving: 2
Preparation Time: 25 Minutes
Cooking Time: 10 Minutes

Ingredients

1 cup uncooked small tube pasta

1 small onion, chopped

1 tablespoon olive oil

2 garlic cloves, minced

1 can (14-1/2 ounces) Italian diced tomatoes

1/2 teaspoon dried basil

1/2 teaspoon dried oregano

1/4 teaspoon sugar

1/4 teaspoon pepper

1/4 cup shredded part-skim mozzarella cheese

1/4 cup grated Parmesan cheese

Direction

Cook pasta according to package directions. In a small saucepan, sauté onion in oil until tender. Add garlic; cook 1 minute longer. Stir in the tomatoes, basil, oregano, sugar and pepper. Bring to a boil. Reduce heat; simmer, uncovered, for 15 minutes. Drain pasta; stir into saucepan.

Transfer to a greased 1-qt. baking dish. Top with cheeses. Bake, uncovered, at 375 degrees for 10-15 minutes or until cheese is melted.

Nutrition:

Calories: 373 calories

Total Fat: 13g

Cholesterol: 16mg

Sodium: 1048mg

Total Carbohydrate: 50g

Protein: 15g

Fiber: 4g

89. Traditional Lasagna

Serving: 12
Preparation Time: 30 Minutes
Cooking Time: 01 h 10 Minutes

Ingredients

1 pound ground beef

3/4 pound Jones No Sugar Pork Sausage Roll sausage

3 cans (8 ounces each) tomato sauce

2 cans (6 ounces each) tomato paste

2 garlic cloves, minced

2 teaspoons sugar

1 teaspoon Italian seasoning

1/2 to 1 teaspoon salt

1/4 to 1/2 teaspoon pepper

3 large eggs

3 tablespoons minced fresh parsley

3 cups 4% small-curd cottage cheese

1 carton (8 ounces) ricotta cheese

1/2 cup grated Parmesan cheese

9 lasagna noodles, cooked and drained

6 slices provolone cheese (about 6 ounces)

3 cups shredded part-skim mozzarella cheese, divided

Direction

In a large skillet over medium heat, cook and crumble beef and sausage until no longer pink; drain. Add next seven ingredients. Bring to a boil. Reduce heat; simmer, uncovered, 1 hour, stirring occasionally. Adjust seasoning with additional salt and pepper, if desired.

Meanwhile, in a large bowl, lightly beat eggs. Add parsley; stir in cottage cheese, ricotta and Parmesan cheese.

Preheat oven to 375 degrees. Spread 1 cup meat sauce in an ungreased 13x9-in. baking dish. Layer with three noodles, provolone cheese, 2 cups cottage cheese mixture, 1 cup mozzarella, three noodles, 2 cups meat sauce, remaining cottage cheese mixture and 1 cup mozzarella. Top with remaining noodles, meat sauce and mozzarella (dish will be full).

Cover; bake 50 minutes. Uncover; bake until heated through, 20 minutes. Let stand 15 minutes before cutting.

Nutrition:

Calories: 503 calories

Total Fat: 27g

Cholesterol: 136mg

Sodium: 1208mg

Total Carbohydrate: 30g

Protein: 36g

Fiber: 2g

90. Tuna N Pea Casserole

Serving: 6
Preparation Time: 20 Minutes
Cooking Time: 40 Minutes

Ingredients

8 ounces uncooked egg noodles

2 cans (10-3/4 ounces each) condensed cream of mushroom soup, undiluted

1/2 cup mayonnaise

1/2 cup 2% milk

2 to 3 teaspoons prepared horseradish

1/2 teaspoon dill weed

1/8 teaspoon pepper

1 cup frozen peas, thawed

1 can (4 ounces) mushroom stems and pieces, drained

1 small onion, chopped

1 jar (2 ounces) diced pimientos, drained

2 cans (6 ounces each) tuna, drained and flaked

1/4 cup dry bread crumbs

1 tablespoon butter, melted

Direction

Cook noodles according to package directions. Meanwhile, in a large bowl, combine the soup, mayonnaise, milk, horseradish, dill and pepper. Stir in the peas, mushrooms, onion, pimientos and tuna.

Drain noodles; stir into soup mixture. Transfer to a greased 2-qt. baking dish. Toss bread crumbs and butter; sprinkle over the top.

Bake, uncovered, at 375 degrees for 40-45 minutes or until bubbly.

Nutrition:

Calories: 505 calories

Total Fat: 25g

Cholesterol: 66mg

Sodium: 1196mg

Total Carbohydrate: 45g

Protein: 24g

Fiber: 5g

91. Tuna Spinach Casserole

Serving: 8
Preparation Time: 25 Minutes
Cooking Time: 50 Minutes

Ingredients

5 cups uncooked egg noodles

2 cups (16 ounces) sour cream

1-1/2 cups mayonnaise

2 to 3 teaspoons lemon juice

2 to 3 teaspoons 2% milk

1/4 teaspoon salt

1 package (10 ounces) frozen chopped spinach, thawed and squeezed dry

1 package (6 ounces) chicken stuffing mix

1/3 cup seasoned bread crumbs

1 can (6 ounces) tuna, drained and flaked

3 tablespoons grated Parmesan cheese

Direction

Cook noodles according to package directions. Meanwhile, in a large bowl, combine the sour cream, mayonnaise, lemon juice, milk and salt. Stir in the spinach, stuffing mix, bread crumbs and tuna until well combined.

Drain noodles and place in a greased 13-in. x 9-in. baking dish. Top with tuna mixture; sprinkle with cheese. Cover and bake at 350 degrees for 45 minutes. Uncover; bake 5-10 minutes longer or until lightly browned and heated through.

Nutrition:

Calories: 673 calories

Total Fat: 46g

Cholesterol: 90mg

Sodium: 927mg

Total Carbohydrate: 42g

Protein: 17g

Fiber: 2g

92. Turkey Alfredo Tetrazzini

Serving: 4
Preparation Time: 20 Minutes
Cooking Time: 30 Minutes

Ingredients

4 ounces thin spaghetti

1 jar (15 ounces) Alfredo sauce

2 cups frozen peas

1-1/2 cups cubed cooked turkey or chicken

1 can (4 ounces) mushroom stems and pieces, drained

1/4 cup shredded Swiss cheese

1/4 cup shredded Parmesan cheese

2 tablespoons white wine or chicken broth

1/2 teaspoon onion powder

1/2 cup french-fried onions

1/2 teaspoon paprika

Direction

Cook spaghetti according to package directions. Meanwhile, in a large bowl, combine the Alfredo sauce, peas, turkey, mushrooms, cheeses, wine and onion powder. Drain spaghetti. Add to sauce mixture; toss to coat. Transfer to a greased 8-in. square baking dish. Sprinkle with onions and paprika.

Cover and bake at 350 degrees until heated through, 30-35 minutes.

Nutrition:

Calories: 504 calories

Total Fat: 21g

Cholesterol: 79mg

Sodium: 808mg

Total Carbohydrate: 44g

Protein: 32g

Fiber: 6g

93. Turkey Florentine

Serving: 6
Preparation Time: 15 Minutes
Cooking Time: 25 Minutes

Ingredients

1 package (10 ounces) frozen chopped spinach

2 tablespoons butter

2 cups cooked noodles

1-1/2 cups diced cooked turkey

1 cup turkey or chicken gravy

1 carton (8 ounces) sour cream onion dip

1/2 teaspoon onion salt

2 tablespoons grated Parmesan cheese

Direction

Cook spinach according to package directions; drain. Stir in butter. Place noodles in a greased 11x7-in. baking dish; top with spinach.

In a large bowl, combine the turkey, gravy, onion dip and onion salt; spoon over spinach. Sprinkle with cheese. Bake, uncovered, at 325 degrees for 25 minutes or until bubbly.

Nutrition:

Calories: 253 calories

Total Fat: 12g

Cholesterol: 60mg

Sodium: 696mg

Total Carbohydrate: 20g

Protein: 16g

Fiber: 2g

94. Turkey Lasagna Rollups

Serving: 4
Preparation Time: 20 Minutes
Cooking Time: 45 Minutes

Ingredients

4 lasagna noodles

6 ounces lean ground turkey

1 small onion, chopped

1 cup chopped fresh broccoli

1/4 cup water

1 cup (8 ounces) reduced-fat ricotta cheese

1 egg, lightly beaten

1 tablespoon fat-free milk

1-1/2 teaspoons minced fresh thyme or 1/2 teaspoon dried thyme

1/4 teaspoon salt

2 cups meatless spaghetti sauce, divided

1/4 cup shredded Parmesan cheese

Direction

Cook the noodles according to package directions; rinse and drain. In a nonstick skillet, cook turkey and onion over medium heat until turkey is no longer pink.

Meanwhile, in a small saucepan, bring broccoli and water to a boil. Reduce heat; cover and simmer for 5 minutes or until crisp-tender; drain.

Add the broccoli, ricotta, egg, milk, thyme and salt to the turkey mixture. Spread over each noodle; drizzle each with 1/4 cup spaghetti sauce. Carefully roll up jelly-roll style.

Place seam side down in an 8-in. square baking dish coated with cooking spray. Drizzle with remaining spaghetti sauce.

Cover and bake at 375 degrees for 45-50 minutes or until a thermometer reads 160 degrees. Sprinkle with Parmesan cheese.

Nutrition:

Calories: 347 calories

Total Fat: 13g

Cholesterol: 110mg

Sodium: 853mg

Total Carbohydrate: 33g

Protein: 23g

Fiber: 4g

95. Turkey Meatball Soup

Serving: 12(3 quarts).
Preparation Time: 30 Minutes
Cooking Time: 10 Minutes

Ingredients

MEATBALLS:

1/4 cup cooked rice

1/4 cup finely chopped onion

1/4 cup finely chopped celery

2 tablespoons all-purpose flour

2 tablespoons water

1/2 teaspoon ground cumin

1/2 teaspoon salt, optional

1/8 teaspoon pepper

3/4 pound ground turkey breast

SOUP:

6 cup chicken broth

1 cup uncooked fine egg noodles

1/2 teaspoon pepper

1/4 teaspoon garlic salt, optional

1/8 teaspoon dill weed

1 tablespoon minced fresh parsley

Direction

In a bowl, combine the first eight ingredients. Add turkey; mix well. Shape into 1-in. balls. Place meatballs on two racks that have coated with cooking spray in shallow baking pans. Bake, uncovered, at 450 degrees for 15 minutes or until turkey is no longer pink; drain. In a Dutch oven or large soup kettle, bring broth to a boil. Add meatballs, noodles, pepper, garlic salt if desired and dill; return to a boil. Reduce heat and simmer, uncovered, for 5 minutes or until noodles are tender. Stir in parsley.

Nutrition:

Calories: 65 calories

Total Fat: 2g

Cholesterol: 19mg

Sodium: 77mg

Total Carbohydrate: 5g

Protein: 9g

Fiber: 0 g

96. Turkey Mushroom Casserole

Serving: 2 casseroles (4each).
Preparation Time: 50 Minutes
Cooking Time: 30 Minutes

Ingredients

1 pound uncooked spaghetti

1/2 pound sliced fresh mushrooms

1 cup chopped onion

2 tablespoons olive oil

1/2 teaspoon minced garlic

3 cans (10-3/4 ounces each) condensed cream of mushroom soup, undiluted

3 cups cubed cooked turkey

1 cup chicken broth

1/3 cup sherry or additional chicken broth

1 teaspoon Italian seasoning

3/4 teaspoon pepper

2 cups grated Parmesan cheese, divided

Direction

Cook spaghetti according to package directions.

Meanwhile, in a Dutch oven, sauté mushrooms and onion in oil until tender. Add the garlic; cook 1 minute longer. Stir in the soup, turkey, broth, sherry, Italian seasoning, pepper and 1 cup cheese. Drain spaghetti; stir into turkey mixture.

Transfer to two greased 8-in. square baking dishes. Sprinkle with remaining cheese. Cover and freeze one casserole for up to 3 months. Cover and bake the remaining casserole at 350 degrees for 30-40 minutes or until heated through.

To use frozen casserole: Thaw in the refrigerator overnight. Remove from the refrigerator 30 minutes before baking. Cover and bake at 350 degrees for 45 minutes. Uncover; bake 5-10 minutes longer or until bubbly.

Nutrition:

Calories: 534 calories

Total Fat: 19g

Cholesterol: 63mg

Sodium: 1286mg

Total Carbohydrate: 55g

Protein: 33g

Fiber: 4g

97. Turkey Mushroom Tetrazzini

Serving: 6
Preparation Time: 25 Minutes
Cooking Time: 25 Minutes

Ingredients

8 ounces uncooked spaghetti

3 tablespoons cornstarch

1 can (14-1/2 ounces) reduced-sodium chicken broth

1/2 teaspoon seasoned salt

Dash pepper

1 tablespoon butter

1/4 cup finely chopped onion

1 garlic clove, minced

1 can (12 ounces) fat-free evaporated milk

2-1/2 cups cubed cooked turkey breast

1 can (4 ounces) mushroom stems and pieces, drained

2 tablespoons grated Parmesan cheese

1/4 teaspoon paprika

Direction

Preheat oven to 350 degrees. Cook spaghetti according to package directions; drain.

Mix cornstarch, broth and seasonings. In a large saucepan, heat butter over medium-high heat; sauté onion until tender. Add garlic; cook and stir 1 minute. Stir cornstarch mixture and add to pan. Bring to a boil; cook and stir until thickened, 1-2 minutes. Reduce heat to low. Add milk; cook and stir 2-3 minutes. Stir in turkey, mushrooms and spaghetti.

Transfer to an 8-in. square baking dish coated with cooking spray. Bake, covered, 20 minutes. Sprinkle with cheese and paprika; bake, uncovered, until heated through, 5-10 minutes.

Nutrition:

Calories: 331 calories

Total Fat: 5g

Cholesterol: 51mg

Sodium: 544mg

Total Carbohydrate: 41g

Protein: 28g

Fiber: 1g

98. Turkey N Squash Lasagna

Serving: 12
Preparation Time: 01 h 10 Minutes
Cooking Time: 50 Minutes

Ingredients

1 medium spaghetti squash (2 to 2-1/2 pounds)

1 pound lean ground turkey

1 large onion, chopped

1 tablespoon olive oil, divided

2 garlic cloves, minced

2 cans (28 ounces each) crushed tomatoes

1 can (6 ounces) tomato paste

1/3 cup minced fresh parsley

1 teaspoon sugar

1 teaspoon dried basil

1 teaspoon dried oregano

1/2 teaspoon salt

1/4 teaspoon pepper

1 egg, lightly beaten

1 carton (15 ounces) reduced-fat ricotta cheese

3/4 cup plus 2 tablespoons grated Parmesan cheese, divided

2 medium zucchini, sliced

6 lasagna noodles, cooked and drained

2 cups shredded part-skim mozzarella cheese, divided

Direction

With a sharp knife, pierce spaghetti squash 10 times. Place on a microwave-safe plate; microwave on high for 5-6 minutes. Turn; cook 4-5 minutes longer or until fork-tender. Cover and let stand for 15 minutes. Cut squash in half lengthwise; discard seeds. Scoop out squash, separating strands with a fork; set aside.

In a large saucepan, cook turkey and onion in 1-1/2 teaspoons oil over medium heat until meat is no longer pink. Add garlic; cook 1 minute longer. Drain. Stir in the tomatoes, tomato paste, parsley, sugar and seasonings. Bring to a boil. Reduce heat; cover and simmer for 30 minutes.

In a small bowl, combine the egg, ricotta and 3/4 cup Parmesan until blended. In a small skillet, sauté zucchini in remaining oil until crisp-tender.

Spread 1-1/2 cups meat sauce into a 13x9-in. baking dish coated with cooking spray. Layer with three noodles and half of the zucchini, spaghetti squash and ricotta mixture. Sprinkle with 1-1/2 cups mozzarella and half of remaining sauce. Top with the remaining noodles, zucchini, spaghetti squash, ricotta mixture and sauce (dish will be full).

Place dish on a baking sheet. Bake, uncovered, at 350 degrees for 45-55 minutes or until edges are bubbly. Sprinkle with remaining mozzarella and Parmesan cheeses. Bake 5 minutes longer or until cheese is melted. Let stand for 10 minutes before cutting.

Nutrition:

Calories: 311 calories

Total Fat: 12g

Cholesterol: 72mg

Sodium: 548mg

Total Carbohydrate: 31g

Protein: 22g

Fiber: 5g

99. Turkey Sausage And Noodles

Serving: 8
Preparation Time: 25 Minutes
Cooking Time: 30 Minutes

Ingredients

2 cups uncooked egg noodles

2 pounds Italian turkey sausage, cut into 1-inch slices

1 large onion, chopped

2 medium carrots, sliced

1/2 cup chopped green pepper

1/2 cup all-purpose flour

2-1/2 cups milk

1/4 cup Worcestershire sauce

1/4 teaspoon rubbed sage

Direction

Cook noodles according to package directions. Meanwhile, in a large skillet, cook the sausage, onion, carrots and green pepper over medium heat until meat is no longer pink. Stir in flour until blended. Gradually add milk. Bring to a boil; cook and stir for 2 minutes or until thickened.

Drain noodles. Add the noodles, Worcestershire sauce and sage to the sausage mixture; toss to coat.

Transfer to a greased 2-1/2-qt. baking dish. Cover and bake at 350 degrees for 20 minutes. Uncover; bake 10-15 minutes longer or until bubbly.

Nutrition:

Calories: 300 calories

Total Fat: 14g

Cholesterol: 87mg

Sodium: 805mg

Total Carbohydrate: 21g

Protein: 23g

Fiber: 1g

100. Turkey Sausage Casserole

Serving: 8
Preparation Time: 15 Minutes
Cooking Time: 20 Minutes

Ingredients

1/2 cup finely chopped onion

2 teaspoons butter, divided

1 pound low-fat smoked turkey sausage, cut into 1/4-inch slices

1 package (10 ounces) spiral noodles, cooked and drained

1/2 pound fresh mushrooms, sliced

1 can (10-3/4 ounces) reduced-fat reduced-sodium condensed cream of chicken soup, undiluted

1 can (10-3/4 ounces) condensed cheddar cheese soup, undiluted

1 cup fat-free evaporated milk

1/2 cup crushed reduced-fat butter-flavored crackers

Direction

In a skillet, sauté onion in 1 teaspoon butter until tender. Add sausage, noodles, mushrooms, soups and milk; mix well. Transfer to a 13-in. x 9-in. baking dish coated with cooking spray. Sprinkle with cracker crumbs; dot with remaining butter.

Bake, uncovered, at 375 degrees for 20-25 minutes or until heated through.

Nutrition:

Calories: 320 calories

Total Fat: 7g

Cholesterol: 29mg

Sodium: 1018mg

Total Carbohydrate: 48g

Protein: 17g

Fiber: 2g

101.   Turkey Spaghetti Casserole

Serving: 6
Preparation Time: 30 Minutes
Cooking Time: 01 h 15 Minutes

Ingredients

1 medium onion, chopped

1 medium carrot, chopped

1 celery rib, chopped

1/3 cup sliced fresh mushrooms

1 tablespoon butter

2-1/2 cups reduced-sodium chicken broth

1 can (10-3/4 ounces) reduced-fat reduced-sodium condensed cream of mushroom soup, undiluted

1/4 teaspoon salt

1/4 teaspoon pepper

2-1/2 cups cubed cooked turkey breast

6 ounces uncooked spaghetti, broken into 2-inch pieces

1/2 cup shredded reduced-fat Colby-Monterey Jack cheese

1/2 teaspoon paprika

Direction

In a small skillet, sauté the vegetables in butter until tender. In a large bowl, combine the broth, soup, salt and pepper.

In a 2-1/2-qt. baking dish coated with cooking spray, layer the turkey, spaghetti and vegetable mixture. Pour broth mixture over the top.

Cover and bake at 350 degrees for 70-80 minutes or until spaghetti is tender, stirring once. Uncover; sprinkle with cheese and paprika. Bake 5-10 minutes longer or until cheese is melted.

Nutrition:

Calories: 284 calories

Total Fat: 6g

Cholesterol: 62mg

Sodium: 702mg

Total Carbohydrate: 30g

Protein: 26g

Fiber: 3g

102.   Turkey Tetrazzini For Two

Serving: 2
Preparation Time: 15 Minutes
Cooking Time: 25 Minutes

Ingredients

2 ounces uncooked spaghetti, broken in half

1 cup cubed cooked turkey breast

2/3 cup condensed cream of chicken soup, undiluted

1/2 cup shredded cheddar cheese

1/3 cup chopped onion

1 tablespoon diced pimientos

1 teaspoon Worcestershire sauce

1/8 teaspoon salt, optional

1 tablespoon grated Parmesan cheese

Direction

Cook spaghetti according to package directions; drain. Stir in the turkey, soup, cheese, onion, pimientos, Worcestershire sauce and salt if desired.

Transfer to a 1-qt. baking dish coated with cooking spray. Sprinkle with Parmesan cheese. Bake, uncovered, at 350 degrees for 25-30 minutes or until bubbly.

Nutrition:

Calories: 361 calories

Total Fat: 9g

Cholesterol: 89mg

Sodium: 617mg

Total Carbohydrate: 33g

Protein: 35g

Fiber: 1g

103.　Twocheese Mac N Cheese

Serving: 15
Preparation Time: 30 Minutes
Cooking Time: 35 Minutes

Ingredients

1 package (16 ounces) spiral pasta

3 tablespoons butter

3 garlic cloves, minced, optional

3 tablespoons all-purpose flour

1/8 teaspoon pepper

Dash salt

4 cups 2% milk

5 cups shredded sharp cheddar cheese, divided

1 cup shredded Asiago cheese

Direction

In a Dutch oven, cook pasta according to package directions.

Meanwhile, in a large saucepan, melt butter over medium heat. Add garlic if desired; cook and stir for 1 minute. Stir in flour, pepper and salt until blended; cook and stir until golden brown, about 5 minutes. Gradually whisk in milk, stirring until smooth. Bring to a boil; cook 2 minutes longer or until thickened.

Remove from heat. Stir in 4 cups cheddar cheese and Asiago cheese until melted. Mixture will thicken.

Preheat oven to 350 degrees. Drain pasta; stir in cheese sauce. Transfer to a greased 13x9-in. baking dish. Sprinkle with remaining cheddar cheese.

Bake, uncovered, 35-40 minutes or until golden brown. Let stand 5 minutes before serving.

Nutrition:

Calories: 331 calories

Total Fat: 17g

Cholesterol: 58mg

Sodium: 306mg

Total Carbohydrate: 28g

Protein: 16g

Fiber: 1g

104.   Twocheese Spaghetti Bake

Serving: 6
Preparation Time: 30 Minutes
Cooking Time: 25 Minutes

Ingredients

6 ounces uncooked spaghetti, broken into thirds

1 pound ground beef

1/4 cup chopped onion

1 jar (14 ounces) spaghetti sauce

2 tablespoons butter

4 teaspoons all-purpose flour

1/4 teaspoon salt

3/4 cup evaporated milk

1/3 cup water

4 ounces process cheese (Velveeta), cubed, divided

2 tablespoons grated Parmesan cheese

Direction

Cook spaghetti according to package directions. Meanwhile, in a large skillet, cook beef and onion over medium heat until meat is no longer pink; drain. Add spaghetti sauce; bring to a boil. Reduce heat; simmer, uncovered, for 10 minutes. Drain spaghetti; stir into beef mixture. Set aside.

In a small saucepan, melt butter. Stir in flour and salt; gradually stir in milk and water. Bring to a boil; cook and stir until thickened and bubbly. Add 1/2 cup process cheese and Parmesan cheese; stir until melted.

Spread half of the spaghetti mixture into a greased 11x7-in. baking dish. Cover with cheese sauce; top with remaining spaghetti mixture and process cheese.

Bake, uncovered, at 350 degrees for 25-30 minutes or until heated through.

Nutrition:

Calories: 409 calories

Total Fat: 19g

Cholesterol: 74mg

Sodium: 829mg

Total Carbohydrate: 36g

Protein: 25g

Fiber: 2g

105.   Twocheese Ziti

Serving: 5
Preparation Time: 25 Minutes
Cooking Time: 25 Minutes

Ingredients

3 cups uncooked ziti or small tube pasta

1 tablespoon butter

2 tablespoons all-purpose flour

1/2 teaspoon salt

1/4 teaspoon pepper

1-3/4 cups fat-free milk

3/4 cup shredded reduced-fat cheddar cheese

2 tablespoons grated Parmesan cheese

TOPPING:

3 tablespoons dry bread crumbs

1-1/2 teaspoons butter, melted

1/4 cup shredded reduced-fat cheddar cheese

3 tablespoons grated Parmesan cheese

Direction

Cook ziti according to package directions. Meanwhile, in a large nonstick skillet, melt butter. Stir in the flour, salt and pepper until smooth; gradually add milk. Bring to a boil; cook and stir for 2 minutes or until thickened. Remove from the heat; stir in cheeses until melted.

Drain ziti; add to sauce and stir to coat. Transfer to a shallow 1-1/2-qt. baking dish coated with cooking spray. Cover and bake at 350 degrees for 20 minutes.

In a small bowl, combine bread crumbs and butter; stir in cheeses. Sprinkle over ziti. Bake, uncovered, for 5-10 minutes or until heated through and topping is lightly browned.

Nutrition:

Calories: 340 calories

Total Fat: 11g

Cholesterol: 31mg

Sodium: 590mg

Total Carbohydrate: 44g

Protein: 18g

Fiber: 2g

106.   Twomeat Macaroni

Serving: 8
Preparation Time: 15 Minutes
Cooking Time: 01 h 30 Minutes

Ingredients

1/2 pound ground beef

1/2 pound ground pork

2 cans (14-1/2 ounces each) diced tomatoes

2 cups shredded cheddar cheese

2 cups uncooked elbow macaroni

1 medium onion, finely chopped

1 cup frozen peas, thawed

2 cans (2-1/2 ounces each) sliced ripe olives, drained

1 jar (2 ounces) diced pimientos, drained

1 teaspoon salt

1/2 teaspoon paprika

1/4 teaspoon celery salt

Direction

In a large skillet, cook beef and pork over medium heat until no longer pink; drain. Add the remaining ingredients.

Transfer to a greased 3-qt. baking dish. Bake, uncovered, at 350 degrees for 1-1/2 hours or until the macaroni is tender, stirring every 30 minutes.

Nutrition:

Calories: 315 calories

Total Fat: 16g

Cholesterol: 63mg

Sodium: 710mg

Total Carbohydrate: 22g

Protein: 20g

Fiber: 3g

107.   Vegetable Noodle Bake

Serving: 4
Preparation Time: 15 Minutes
Cooking Time: 20 Minutes

Ingredients

1 can (14-1/2 ounces) diced tomatoes, drained

3/4 cup canned tomato puree

1/3 cup chopped onion

1-1/4 teaspoons dried oregano

1/4 teaspoon garlic powder

1/4 teaspoon salt

1/8 teaspoon pepper

2-1/2 cups uncooked medium egg noodles

1/2 cup 4% cottage cheese

1 package (10 ounces) frozen chopped spinach, thawed and squeezed dry

1/3 cup shredded American cheese

Direction

In a large saucepan, combine the tomatoes, tomato puree, onion, oregano, garlic powder, salt and pepper. Bring to a boil. Reduce heat; simmer, uncovered, for 15 minutes.

Meanwhile, cook noodles according to package directions; drain.

Spread 1/3 cup tomato mixture in a greased shallow 2-qt. baking dish. Top with half of the noodles. Spread with cottage cheese; top with spinach. Drizzle with 1/2 cup tomato mixture; top with remaining noodles and tomato mixture. Sprinkle with American cheese. Cover and bake at 350 degrees for 20-25 minutes or until cheese is melted.

Nutrition:

Calories: 211 calories

Total Fat: 5g

Cholesterol: 35mg

Sodium: 559mg

Total Carbohydrate: 31g

Protein: 12g

Fiber: 5g

108. Vegetable Tuna Noodle Casserole

Serving: 4-6
Preparation Time: 35 Minutes
Cooking Time: 25 Minutes

Ingredients

3 cups uncooked egg noodles

1 cup chopped celery

1/3 cup chopped onion

1/4 cup chopped green pepper

1 tablespoon canola oil

1 can (10-3/4 ounces) condensed cream of mushroom soup, undiluted

1 cup shredded cheddar cheese

1 cup whole milk

1 can (12 ounces) tuna, drained and flaked

1/2 cup mayonnaise

1 jar (2 ounces) diced pimientos, drained

1/2 teaspoon salt

Direction

Cook noodles according to package directions. Meanwhile, in a skillet, sauté the celery, onion and green pepper in oil until tender; set aside. In a saucepan, combine the soup, cheese and milk. Cook and stir over low heat until cheese is melted.

Drain noodles; place in a large bowl. Add the celery mixture, soup mixture, tuna, mayonnaise, pimientos and salt. Pour into a greased 8-in. square baking dish. Bake, uncovered, at 350 degrees for 25-30 minutes or until heated through.

Nutrition:

Calories: 435 calories

Total Fat: 27g

Cholesterol: 69mg

Sodium: 1001mg

Total Carbohydrate: 23g

Protein: 24g

Fiber: 2g

109. Veggie Couscous Quiche

Serving: 6
Preparation Time: 25 Minutes
Cooking Time: 50 Minutes

Ingredients

1 large egg

1/2 teaspoon onion salt

2 cups cooked couscous, cooled

1/4 cup shredded Swiss cheese

FILLING:

4 large eggs

1 cup half-and-half cream

4 cups frozen broccoli florets, thawed

1 can (6 ounces) sliced mushrooms, drained

1 cup shredded Swiss cheese, divided

1/4 teaspoon ground nutmeg

1 plum tomato, finely chopped

2 green onions, chopped

Direction

In a large bowl, whisk egg and onion salt. Add couscous and cheese; stir until blended. Press onto the bottom and up the sides of a greased 9-in. deep-dish pie plate. Bake at 350 degrees for 5 minutes.

For filling, in a large bowl, whisk eggs and cream. Stir in the broccoli, mushrooms, 1/2 cup cheese and nutmeg. Pour into crust. Bake for 45-55 minutes or until a knife inserted in the center comes out clean.

Sprinkle with tomato, onions and remaining cheese. Bake 3-5 minutes longer or until cheese is melted. Let stand for 10 minutes before cutting.

Nutrition:

Calories: 281 calories

Total Fat: 15g

Cholesterol: 217mg

Sodium: 423mg

Total Carbohydrate: 19g

Protein: 17g

Fiber: 3g

110.   Very Veggie Lasagna

Serving: 12
Preparation Time: 40 Minutes
Cooking Time: 60 Minutes

Ingredients

2 medium carrots, julienned

1 medium zucchini, cut into 1/4-inch slices

1 yellow summer squash, cut into 1/4-inch slices

1 medium onion, sliced

1 cup fresh broccoli florets

1/2 cup sliced celery

1/2 cup julienned sweet red pepper

1/2 cup julienned green pepper

1/2 to 1 teaspoon salt

2 tablespoons canola oil

2 garlic cloves, minced

3-1/2 cups spaghetti sauce

14 lasagna noodles, cooked and drained

4 cups shredded part-skim mozzarella cheese

Direction

In a large skillet, stir-fry vegetables and salt in oil until crisp-tender. Add garlic; cook 1 minute longer.

Spread 3/4 cup spaghetti sauce in the greased 13x9-in. baking dish. Arrange seven noodles over sauce, overlapping as needed. Layer with half of the vegetables, spaghetti sauce and cheese. Repeat layers.

Cover and bake at 350 degrees for 60-65 minutes or until bubbly. Let stand for 15 minutes before cutting.

Nutrition:

Calories: 295 calories

Total Fat: 11g

Cholesterol: 23mg

Sodium: 617mg

Total Carbohydrate: 34g

Protein: 16g

Fiber: 3g

111.   Weeknight Lazy Lasagna

Serving: 6
Preparation Time: 20 Minutes
Cooking Time: 10 Minutes

Ingredients

8 ounces uncooked lasagna noodles, broken into 2-inch pieces

1 cup part-skim ricotta cheese

1 cup shredded part-skim mozzarella cheese, divided

1/3 cup grated Parmesan cheese

1 jar (24 ounces) pasta sauce with meat

Direction

Preheat oven to 400 degrees. Cook lasagna noodles according to package directions. Meanwhile, in a large bowl, mix ricotta cheese, 1/2 cup mozzarella cheese and Parmesan cheese. Drain noodles well; stir into cheese mixture.

Spread 1 cup pasta sauce into a greased 11x7-in. baking dish. Layer with half of the noodle mixture and 1 cup sauce; layer with the remaining noodle mixture and sauce. Sprinkle with remaining cheese.

Cover with greased foil; bake until heated through, 10-15 minutes.

Nutrition:

Calories: 332 calories

Total Fat: 10g

Cholesterol: 29mg

Sodium: 901mg

Total Carbohydrate: 45g

Protein: 17g

Fiber: 3g

112. Wheres The Squash Lasagna

Serving: 12
Preparation Time: 40 Minutes
Cooking Time: 60 Minutes

Ingredients

1 pound ground beef

2 large zucchini (about 1 pound), shredded

3/4 cup chopped onion

2 garlic cloves, minced

1 can (14-1/2 ounces) stewed tomatoes

2 cups water

1 can (12 ounces) tomato paste

1 tablespoon minced fresh parsley

1-1/2 teaspoons salt

1 teaspoon sugar

1/2 teaspoon dried oregano

1/2 teaspoon pepper

9 lasagna noodles, cooked, rinsed and drained

1 carton (15 ounces) ricotta cheese

2 cups shredded part-skim mozzarella cheese

1 cup grated Parmesan cheese

Direction

In a skillet, cook the beef, zucchini and onion over medium heat until meat is no longer pink. Add garlic; cook 1 minute longer. Drain.

Place tomatoes in a food processor or blender; cover and process until smooth. Stir into beef mixture. Add the water, tomato paste, parsley and seasonings. Bring to a boil. Reduce heat; simmer, uncovered, for 30 minutes, stirring occasionally.

Spread 1 cup meat sauce in a greased 13x9-in. baking dish. Arrange three noodles over sauce. Spread with a third of the meat sauce; top with half of the ricotta cheese. Sprinkle with a third of the mozzarella and Parmesan cheeses. Repeat. Top with remaining noodles, meat sauce and cheeses.

Cover and bake at 350 degrees for 45 minutes. Uncover; bake 15 minutes longer or until bubbly. Let stand for 15 minutes before cutting.

Nutrition:

Calories: 309 calories

Total Fat: 13g

Cholesterol: 53mg

Sodium: 642mg

Total Carbohydrate: 27g

Protein: 21g

Fiber: 3g

113. Whole Wheat Pasta Bake

Serving: 4
Preparation Time: 10 Minutes
Cooking Time: 15 Minutes

Ingredients

2 cups uncooked whole wheat spiral pasta

1/2 pound boneless skinless chicken breasts, cubed

3 tablespoons butter, divided

1 medium zucchini, chopped

1/4 cup chopped onion

2 tablespoons all-purpose flour

1-1/2 cups half-and-half cream

3/4 pound process cheese (Velveeta), cubed

1/2 teaspoon Italian seasoning

TOPPING:

1 cup dry whole wheat bread crumbs

3 tablespoons butter, melted

1/2 teaspoon Italian seasoning

1/4 teaspoon salt

Direction

Cook pasta according to package directions. Meanwhile, in a large skillet, sauté chicken in 1 tablespoon butter until no longer pink. Remove and keep warm.

In the same skillet, sauté zucchini and onion in remaining butter. Stir in flour until blended; gradually add cream. Bring to a boil; cook and stir for 2 minutes or until thickened. Reduce heat. Stir in cheese and Italian seasoning until cheese is melted; add chicken.

Drain pasta; add to cheese mixture. Transfer to a greased 8-in. square baking dish. In a small bowl, combine the bread crumbs, butter, Italian seasoning and salt; sprinkle over top. Bake, uncovered, at 350 degrees for 10-15 minutes or until heated through and topping is golden brown.

Nutrition:

Calories: 849 calories

Total Fat: 50g

Cholesterol: 190mg

Sodium: 1582mg

Total Carbohydrate: 60g

Protein: 39g

Fiber: 7g

114. Ziti Bake

Serving: 6
Preparation Time: 20 Minutes
Cooking Time: 50 Minutes

Ingredients

3 cups uncooked ziti or small tube pasta

1-3/4 cups meatless spaghetti sauce, divided

1 cup 4% cottage cheese

1-1/2 cups shredded part-skim mozzarella cheese, divided

1 large egg, lightly beaten

2 teaspoons dried parsley flakes

1/2 teaspoon dried oregano

1/4 teaspoon garlic powder

1/8 teaspoon pepper

Direction

Cook pasta according to package directions. Meanwhile, in a large bowl, combine 3/4 cup spaghetti sauce, cottage cheese, 1 cup mozzarella cheese, egg, parsley, oregano, garlic powder and pepper. Drain pasta; stir into cheese mixture.

In a greased 8-in. square baking dish, spread 1/4 cup spaghetti sauce. Top with pasta mixture, remaining sauce and mozzarella cheese.

Cover and bake at 375 degrees for 45 minutes. Uncover; bake 5-10 minutes longer or until a thermometer reads 160 degrees.

Nutrition:

Calories: 289 calories

Total Fat: 8g

Cholesterol: 60mg

Sodium: 616mg

Total Carbohydrate: 37g

Protein: 18g

Fiber: 3g

115.   Ziti Lasagna

Serving: 3
Preparation Time: 15 Minutes
Cooking Time: 20 Minutes

Ingredients

2 cups uncooked ziti or small tube pasta

1/2 pound lean ground beef

1/4 cup chopped onion

1/4 cup chopped green pepper

1 can (8 ounces) tomato sauce

1/2 teaspoon Italian seasoning

1/4 teaspoon garlic powder

Dash pepper

3/4 cup ricotta cheese

1 cup shredded part-skim mozzarella cheese

Direction

Cook ziti according to package directions. Meanwhile, in a skillet, cook the beef, onion and green pepper over medium heat until meat is no longer pink; drain. Stir in the tomato sauce, Italian seasoning, garlic powder and pepper. Cook and stir until heated through, about 3 minutes.

Drain pasta. Spread half of the meat sauce in a 1-qt. baking dish coated with cooking spray. Top with half of the ziti, ricotta cheese and mozzarella cheese. Repeat layers. Bake, uncovered, at 350 degrees for 20-25 minutes or until heated through. Let stand for 5 minutes before serving.

Nutrition:

Calories: 437 calories

Total Fat: 15g

Cholesterol: 83mg

Sodium: 613mg

Total Carbohydrate: 38g

Protein: 35g

Fiber: 2g

116.　Zucchini Pasta Bake

Serving: 2
Preparation Time: 20 Minutes
Cooking Time: 10 Minutes

Ingredients

1 cup diced zucchini

1/2 cup diced green pepper

1/2 cup diced sweet red pepper

1/4 cup diced onion

2 tablespoons vegetable oil

1/4 cup dry bread crumbs

1/4 teaspoon salt-free seasoning blend

1/8 teaspoon pepper

1 cup cooked tricolor spiral pasta

2 tablespoons nonfat Parmesan cheese topping

Direction

In a small skillet, sauté vegetables in oil until tender, about 7 minutes. Stir in the bread crumbs, salt and pepper; cook for 2-3 minutes. Remove from the heat; stir in pasta. Pour into a greased 1-qt. baking dish. Sprinkle with cheese topping. Bake, uncovered, at 375 degrees for 10 minutes or until heated through.

Nutrition:

Calories: 277 calories

Total Fat: 10g

Cholesterol: 5mg

Sodium: 238mg

Total Carbohydrate: 38g

Protein: 9g

Fiber: 4g

117.   Zucchini Pasta Casserole

Serving: 2
Preparation Time: 20 Minutes
Cooking Time: 10 Minutes

Ingredients

1 cup diced zucchini

1/2 cup diced green pepper

1/2 cup diced sweet red pepper

1/4 cup diced onion

2 tablespoons vegetable oil

1/4 cup Italian-seasoned dry bread crumbs

1/4 teaspoon salt

1/8 teaspoon pepper

1 cup cooked tricolor spiral pasta

Grated Parmesan cheese, optional

Direction

In a small skillet, sauté vegetables in oil until tender, about 7 minutes. Stir in the bread crumbs, salt and pepper; cook for 2-3 minutes. Remove from the heat; stir in pasta. Pour into a greased 1-qt. baking dish. Sprinkle with Parmesan cheese if desired. Bake, uncovered, at 375 degrees for 10 minutes or until heated through.

Nutrition:

Calories: 305 calories

Total Fat: 15g

Cholesterol: 1mg

Sodium: 668mg

Total Carbohydrate: 37g

Protein: 7g

Fiber: 0 g

118.   Pesto Parmesan Pork With Green Pasta

Basil, pine nuts and lots of olive oil is excellent for any pasta dish. I love this combo!

Preparation Time: 1 hour 27 minutes
Servings: 4

Ingredients

4 boneless pork chops

Salt and black pepper to taste

½ cup basil pesto, olive oil-based

1 cup grated Parmesan cheese

1 tbsp butter

4 large turnips, spiralized

Directions

Preheat the oven to 350 F.

Season the pork with salt, black pepper and place on a baking sheet. Divide the pesto on top and spread well on the pork.

Place the sheet in the oven and bake for 45 minutes to 1 hour or until cooked through.

When ready, pull out the baking sheet and divide half of the Parmesan cheese on top of the pork. Cook further for 10 minutes or until the cheese melts. Remove the pork and set aside for serving.

Melt the butter in a medium skillet and sauté the turnips until tender, 5 to 7 minutes. Stir in the remaining Parmesan cheese and divide between serving plates.

Top with the pork and serve warm.

Nutrition:

Calories 532; Fats 28.4g; Net Carbs 4.9g; Protein 53.8g

119.   Pork Lo Mein

Are you up for more Asian flavors? This pasta-veggie mix is one to have frequently.

Preparation Time: 25 minutes
Servings: 4

Ingredients

For the keto pasta:

1 cup shredded mozzarella cheese

1 egg yolk

For the pork and vegetables:

1 tbsp sesame oil

3 boneless pork chops, cut into ¼-inch strips

Salt and black pepper to taste

1 red bell pepper, deseeded and thinly sliced

1 yellow bell pepper, deseeded and thinly sliced

1 cup green beans, trimmed and halved

1 garlic clove, minced

1-inch ginger knob, peeled and grated

4 green onions, chopped

1 tsp toasted sesame seeds to garnish

For the sauce:

3 tbsp coconut aminos

2 tsp sesame oil

2 tsp sugar-free maple syrup

1 tsp fresh ginger paste

Directions

For the pasta:

Pour the cheese into a medium safe-microwave bowl and melt in the microwave for 2 minutes while stirring at 20-second intervals until fully melted.

Take out the bowl and allow cooling for 1 minute only to warm the cheese but not cool completely. Mix in the egg yolk until well-combined.

Lay a parchment paper on a flat surface, pour the cheese mixture on top and cover with another parchment paper. Using a rolling pin, flatten the dough into 1/8-inch thickness. Take off the parchment paper and cut the dough into thin spaghetti strands. Place in a bowl and refrigerate overnight.

When ready to cook, bring 2 cups of water to a boil in medium saucepan and add the pasta. Cook for 40 seconds to 1 minute and then drain through a colander. Run cold water over the pasta and set aside to cool.

For the pork and vegetables:

Heat the sesame oil in a large skillet, season the pork with salt, black pepper, and sear in the oil on both sides until brown, 5 minutes. Transfer to a plate and set aside.

Mix in the bell peppers, green beans and cook until sweaty, 3 minutes. Stir in the garlic, ginger, green onions and cook until fragrant, 1 minute.

Add the pork and pasta to the skillet and toss well.

In a small bowl, toss the sauce's ingredients the coconut aminos, sesame oil, maple syrup, and ginger paste.

Pour the mixture over the pork mixture and toss well; cook for 1 minute.

Dish the food onto serving plates and garnish with the sesame seeds. Serve warm.

Nutrition:

Calories 338; Fats 12.6g; Net Carbs 4.6g; Protein 43g

120.   Pasta & Cheese Pulled Pork

Now, this looks more like a regular mac and cheese but tastier and healthier than the traditional type.

Preparation Time: 1 hour 45 minutes
Servings: 4

Ingredients

For the keto macaroni:

1 cup shredded mozzarella cheese

1 egg yolk

For the pulled pork mac and cheese:

2 tbsp olive oil

1 lb pork shoulders, divided into 3 pieces

Salt and black pepper to taste

1 tsp dried thyme

1 cup chicken broth

2 tbsp butter

2 medium shallots, minced

2 garlic cloves, minced

1 cup water

1 cup grated Monterey Jack cheese

4 oz cream cheese, room temperature

1 cup heavy cream

½ tsp white pepper

½ tsp nutmeg powder

2 tbsp chopped parsley

Directions

For the keto macaroni:

Pour the cheese into a medium safe-microwave bowl and melt in the microwave for 2 minutes while stirring at 20-second intervals until fully melted.

Take out the bowl and allow cooling for 1 minute only to warm the cheese but not cool completely. Mix in the egg yolk until well-combined.

Lay a parchment paper on a flat surface, pour the cheese mixture on top and cover with another parchment paper. Using a rolling pin, flatten the dough into 1/8-inch thickness.

Take off the parchment paper and cut the dough into small cubes of the size of macaroni. Place in a bowl and refrigerate overnight.

When ready to cook, bring 2 cups of water to a boil in medium saucepan and add the keto macaroni. Cook for 40 seconds to 1 minute and then drain through a colander. Run cold water over the pasta and set aside to cool.

For the pulled pork mac and cheese:

Heat the olive oil in a large pot, season the pork with salt, black pepper, thyme, and sear in the oil on both sides until brown. Pour on the chicken broth, cover, and cook over low heat for 45 minutes to 1 hour or until softened. When ready, remove the pork onto a plate and shred into small strands. Set aside.

Preheat the oven to 380 F.

Melt the butter in a large skillet and sauté the shallots until softened. Stir in the garlic and cook until fragrant, 30 seconds.

Pour in the water to deglaze the pot and then stir in half of the Monterey Jack cheese and cream cheese until melted, 4 minutes. Mix in the heavy cream and season with salt, black pepper, white pepper, and nutmeg powder.

Add the pasta, pork, and half of the parsley to the mixture; combine well.

Pour the mixture into a baking dish and cover the top with the remaining Monterey Jack cheese. Bake in the oven until the cheese melts and the food bubbly, 15 to 20 minutes.

Remove from the oven, allow cooling for 2 minutes and garnish with the parsley.

Serve warm.

Nutrition:

Calories 603; Fats 43.6g; Net Carbs 1.5g; Protein 45.9g

121.   Creamy Pork With Green Beans And Keto Fettuccine

Preparation Time: 40 minutes

Servings: 4

Ingredients

For the keto fettuccine:

1 cup shredded mozzarella cheese

1 egg yolk

For the creamy pork and green beans:

1 tbsp olive oil

4 pork loin medallions, cut into thin strips

Salt and black pepper to taste

½ cup green beans, chopped

1 lemon, zested and juiced

¼ cup chicken broth

1 cup crème fraiche

6 basil leaves, chopped

1 cup shaved Parmesan cheese for topping

Directions

For the keto fettucine:

Pour the cheese into a medium safe-microwave bowl and melt in the microwave for 2 minutes while stirring at 20-second intervals until fully melted. Take out the bowl and allow cooling for 1 minute only to warm the cheese but not cool completely. Mix in the egg yolk until well-combined.

Lay a parchment paper on a flat surface, pour the cheese mixture on top and cover with another parchment paper. Using a rolling pin, flatten the dough into 1/8-inch thickness. Take off the parchment paper and cut the dough into thick fettuccine strands. Place in a bowl and refrigerate overnight. Bring 2 cups of water to a boil in a saucepan and add keto fettuccine. Cook for 1 minute and then drain. Set aside to cool.

For the creamy pork and green beans:

Heat olive oil in a skillet, season the pork with salt, pepper, and cook for 10 minutes. Mix in green beans and cook for 5 minutes. Stir in lemon zest, lemon juice, and chicken broth. Cook for 5 more minutes or until the liquid reduces by a quarter. Add crème fraiche and mix well. Pour in pasta and basil and cook for 1 minute. Top with Parmesan.

Nutrition:

Calories 586; Fats 32.3g; Net Carbs 9g; Protein 59g

122.   Delicious Sambal Pork Noodles

Preparation Time: 60 minutes
Servings: 4

Ingredients

For the shirataki noodles:

2 (8 oz) packs Miracle noodles, garlic and herb

Salt to season

For the sambal pork:

1 tbsp olive oil

1 lb ground pork

4 garlic cloves, minced

1-inch ginger, peeled and grated

1 tsp liquid stevia

1 tbsp sugar-free tomato paste

2 fresh basil leaves + extra for garnishing

2 tbsp sambal oelek

2 tbsp plain vinegar

1 cup water

2 tbsp coconut aminos

Salt to taste

1 tbsp unsalted butter

Directions

For the shirataki noodles:

Bring 2 cups of water to a boil in a pot over medium heat. Strain the Miracle noodles and rinse very well under hot running water. Allow proper draining and pour the noodles into the boiling water. Take off the heat and let sit for 3 minutes and strain again.

Place a dry skillet over medium heat and stir-fry the shirataki noodles until visibly dry, 1 to 2 minutes. Season with salt, plate and set aside.

For the pork sambal:

Heat the olive oil in a large pot and cook in the pork until brown, 5 minutes. Stir in the garlic, ginger, liquid stevia and cook for 1 minute. Add in tomato paste, cook for 2 minutes and mix in basil, sambal oelek, vinegar, water, coconut aminos, and salt. Cover the pot and continue cooking for 30 minutes. Uncover, add the shirataki noodles, butter and mix well into the sauce. Garnish with some basil leaves and serve warm.

Nutrition:

Calories 505; Fats 30.2g; Net Carbs 22.1g; Protein 33.9g

123.   Lemongrass Pork With Spaghetti Squash

Preparation Time: 1 hour + marinating time
Servings: 4

Ingredients

For the lemongrass pork:

2 tbsp minced lemongrass

2 tbsp fresh ginger paste

2 tbsp sugar-free maple syrup

2 tbsp coconut aminos

1 tbsp fish sauce

4 boneless pork chops

2 tbsp peanut oil

For the squash noodles:

3 lb spaghetti squashes, halved and deseeded

1 tbsp olive oil

Salt and black pepper to taste

For the steamed spinach:

1 tbsp peanut oil

1 tsp fresh ginger paste

1 lb baby spinach

For the peanut-coconut sauce:

½ cup coconut milk

¼ cup organic peanut butter

Directions

For the lemongrass pork:

In a medium bowl, mix the lemongrass, ginger paste, maple syrup, coconut aminos, and fish sauce. Place the pork in the liquid and coat well. Allow marinating for 45 minutes.

After, heat the peanut oil in a large skillet, remove the pork from the marinade and sear in the oil on both sides until golden brown and cooked through, 10 to 15 minutes. Transfer to a plate and cover with foil.

For the spaghetti squash:

Preheat the oven to 380 F.

Place the spaghetti squashes on a baking sheet, brush with the olive oil and season with salt and black pepper. Bake in the oven for 20 to 25 minutes or until tender.

When ready, remove the squash and shred with two forks into spaghetti-like strands. Keep warm in the oven.

For the spinach:

In another skillet, heat the peanut oil and sauté the ginger until fragrant. Add the spinach and cook to wilt while stirring to be coated well in the ginger, 2 minutes.

For the peanut-coconut sauce:

In a medium bowl, quickly whisk the coconut milk with the peanut butter until well combined.

To serve:

Unwrap and divide the pork into four bowls, add the spaghetti squash to the side, then the spinach and drizzle the peanut sauce on top.

Serve immediately.

Nutrition:

Calories 694; Fats 34.1g; Net Carbs 37.1g; Protein 53.6g

124.   Pork Avocado Keto Noodles

Preparation Time: 15 minutes
Servings: 4

Ingredients

2 tbsp butter

1 lb ground pork

Salt and black pepper to taste

8 red and yellow bell peppers, spiralized

1 tsp garlic powder

2 medium avocados, pitted, peeled and mashed

2 tbsp chopped pecans for topping

Directions

Melt the butter in a large skillet and cook the pork until brown, 5 minutes. Season with salt and black pepper. Stir in the bell peppers, garlic powder and cook until the peppers are slightly tender, 2 minutes.

Mix in the mashed avocados, adjust the taste with salt and black pepper and cook for 1 minute. Dish the food onto serving plates, garnish with the pecans and serve warm.

Nutrition:

Calories 704; Fats 49.5g; Net Carbs 22.3g; Protein 35.8g

125.   Chinese Pork And Celeriac Noodles

Preparation Time: 1 hour 18 minutes

Servings: 4

Ingredients

3 tbsp sugar-free maple syrup

3 tbsp coconut aminos

1 tbsp fresh ginger paste

¼ tsp Chinese five spice powder

Salt and black pepper to taste

1 lb pork tenderloin, cut into 1-inch cubes

2 tbsp butter

4 medium large celeriac, spiralized

1 tbsp sesame oil

4 heads baby bok choy, leaves separated

2 green onions, chopped for garnishing

2 tbsp sesame seeds for garnishing

Directions

Preheat the oven to 400 F and line a baking sheet with foil.

In a large bowl, mix the maple syrup, coconut aminos, ginger paste, Chinese five-spice powder, salt, and black pepper. Spoon 3 tablespoons of the mixture into a small bowl and reserve for topping. Mix the pork cubes into the remaining marinade and set aside to marinate for 25 minutes.

Meanwhile, melt the butter in a medium skillet and sauté the celeriac until softened, 5 to 7 minutes or until tender. Turn the heat off and set aside.

When the marinating is over, remove the pork from the marinade onto the baking sheet and cook in the oven for 40 minutes or until cooked through.

When the pork is almost ready, heat the sesame oil in a large skillet and sauté the bok choy and zucchini pasta until slightly wilted and tender, 2 to 3 minutes.

Transfer to serving bowls and top with the pork when ready. Garnish with the green onions and sesame seeds. Drizzle the reserved marinade on top and serve warm.

Nutrition:

Calories 409; Fats 17.8g; Net Carbs 3g; Protein 44.5g

126.   Garlic Pecorino Kohlrabi With Sausage

Preparation Time: 15 minutes
Servings: 4

Ingredients

2 tbsp olive oil

1 cup sliced pork sausage

4 bacon slices, chopped

4 large kohlrabi, spiralized

6 garlic cloves, minced

1 cup cherry tomatoes, halved

Salt and black pepper to taste

7 fresh basil leaves

1 cup grated Pecorino Romano cheese

1 tbsp pine nuts for topping

Directions

Heat the olive oil in a large skillet and cook the sausage and bacon until brown, 5 minutes. Transfer to a plate and set aside.

Stir in the kohlrabi and cook until tender, 5 to 7 minutes. Mix the garlic into the oil and cook until fragrant, 30 seconds. Then, add the cherry tomatoes, salt, and black pepper; cook for 2 minutes.

Mix in the sausage, bacon, basil, and half of the Pecorino Romano cheese. Turn the heat off.

Dish the food onto serving plates and garnish with the remaining cheese and pine nuts.

Serve warm.

Nutrition:

Calories 229; Fats 20.2g; Net Carbs 2.43g; Protein 7.6g

CHICKEN

127.   Chicken Alfredo Zoodles

Preparation Time: 23 minutes
Servings: 4

Ingredients

4 tbsp butter

4 boneless chicken breasts, cut into 1-inch cubes

Salt and black pepper to taste

4 large turnips, spiralized

3 garlic cloves, minced

¾ cup heavy cream

1 cup grated Pecorino Romano cheese

2 tbsp chopped fresh parsley

Directions

Melt 2 tablespoons of butter in a large skillet, season the chicken with salt, black pepper, and cook in the oil until golden brown on both sides and cooked within, 10 minutes. Transfer to a plate and set aside.

Melt the remaining butter in the skillet and sauté the turnips until softened, 6 minutes.

Add the garlic to the pan and cook until fragrant, 1 minute.

Reduce the heat to low and stir in the heavy cream and Pecorino Romano cheese until melted. Season with salt, black pepper.

Stir in the chicken and dish the food onto serving plates.

Garnish with the parsley and serve warm.

Nutrition:

Calories 771; Fats 49.2g; Net Carbs 2.3g; Protein 68.6g

128.   One-Pot Spicy Cheddar Pasta

Preparation Time: 35 minutes

Servings: 4

Ingredients

For the shirataki fettuccine:

2 (8 oz) packs shirataki fettuccine

For the spicy cheddar pasta:

4 chicken breasts

1 medium yellow onion, minced

3 garlic cloves, minced

1 tsp Italian seasoning

½ tsp garlic powder

¼ tsp red chili flakes

¼ tsp cayenne pepper

1 cup sugar-free marinara sauce

1 cup grated mozzarella cheese

½ cup grated cheddar cheese

Salt and black pepper to taste

2 tbsp chopped parsley

Directions

For the shirataki fettuccine:

Boil 2 cups of water in a medium pot over medium heat. Strain the shirataki pasta and rinse very well under hot running water. Allow proper draining and pour the shirataki pasta into the boiling water. Take off the heat and let sit for 3 minutes and strain again.

Place a dry skillet over medium heat and stir-fry the shirataki pasta until visibly dry, and makes a squeaky sound when stirred, 1 to 2 minutes. Take off the heat and set aside.

For the spicy cheddar pasta:

Heat the olive oil in a large pot, season the chicken with salt, black pepper, and cook in the oil until golden brown on both sides and cooked within, 10 minutes. Transfer to a plate, cut into cubes and set aside. Add the onion and garlic to the pan and cook until softened and fragrant, 3 minutes. Season with the Italian seasoning, garlic powder, red chili flakes, and cayenne pepper. Cook for 1 minute.

Stir in marinara sauce and simmer for 5 minutes. Adjust the taste with salt and black pepper. Reduce heat to low and return the chicken to the sauce and shirataki fettucine, mozzarella and cheddar cheeses. Stir until the cheese melts. Garnish with parsley.

Nutrition:

Calories 763; Fats 34g; Net Carbs 17.9g; Protein 82.7g

129. Creamy Tuscan Chicken Linguine

Preparation Time: 35 minutes

Servings: 4

Ingredients

For the keto linguine:

1 cup shredded mozzarella cheese

1 egg yolk

For the creamy Tuscan chicken:

2 tbsp olive oil

4 chicken breasts

1 medium white onion, chopped

1 cup sundried tomatoes in oil, drained and chopped

1 red bell pepper, deseeded and chopped

5 garlic cloves, minced

1 tsp dried oregano

¾ cup chicken broth

1 ½ cup heavy cream

¾ cup grated Pecorino Romano cheese

1 cup baby kale, chopped

Salt and black pepper to taste

Directions

For the keto linguine:

Pour the cheese into a medium safe-microwave bowl and melt in the microwave for 2 minutes while stirring at 20-second intervals until fully melted. Take out the bowl and allow cooling for 1 minute only to warm the cheese but not cool completely. Mix in the egg yolk until well-combined.

Lay a parchment paper on a flat surface, pour the cheese mixture on top and cover with another parchment paper. Using a rolling pin, flatten the dough into 1/8-inch thickness.

Take off the parchment paper and cut the dough into linguine-like strands. Place in a bowl and refrigerate overnight.

When ready to cook, bring 2 cups of water to a boil in medium saucepan and add the keto linguine. Cook for 40 seconds to 1 minute and then drain through a colander. Run cold water over the pasta and set aside to cool.

For the creamy Tuscan chicken:

Heat the olive oil in a large skillet, season the chicken with salt, black pepper, and cook in the oil until golden brown on the outside and cooked within, 7 to 8 minutes. Transfer the chicken to a plate and cut into 4 slices each. Set aside.

Add the onion, sundried tomatoes, bell pepper to the skillet and sauté until softened, 5 minutes. Mix in the garlic, oregano and cook until fragrant, 1 minute.

Deglaze the skillet with the chicken broth and mix in the heavy cream. Simmer for 2 minutes and stir in the Pecorino Romano cheese until melted, 2 minutes.

Once the cheese melts, stir in the kale to wilt and adjust the taste with salt and black pepper.

Mix in the linguine and chicken until well coated in the sauce.

Dish the food and serve warm.

Nutrition:

Calories 941; Fats 60.7g; Net Carbs 10.7g; Protein 79.3g

130.   Tomato Kale Chicken Skillet With Keto Linguine

Preparation Time: 30 minutes

Servings: 4

Ingredients

For the keto linguine:

1 cup shredded mozzarella cheese

1 egg yolk

For the tomato-kale chicken:

3 tbsp olive oil

4 chicken thighs, cut into 1-inch pieces

Salt and black pepper to taste

1 yellow onion, chopped

4 garlic cloves, minced

1 cup cherry tomatoes, halved

½ cup chicken broth

2 cups baby kale, chopped

1 cup grated Parmigiano-Reggiano cheese for serving

2 tbsp pine nuts for topping

Directions

For the keto linguine:

Pour the cheese into a medium safe-microwave bowl and melt in the microwave for 2 minutes while stirring at 20-second intervals until fully melted.

Take out the bowl and allow cooling for 1 minute only to warm the cheese but not cool completely. Mix in the egg yolk until well-combined.

Lay a parchment paper on a flat surface, pour the cheese mixture on top and cover with another parchment paper. Using a rolling pin, flatten the dough into 1/8-inch thickness.

Take off the parchment paper and cut the dough into linguine strands. Place in a bowl and refrigerate overnight.

When ready to cook, bring 2 cups of water to a boil in medium saucepan and add the keto linguine. Cook for 40 seconds to 1 minute and then drain through a colander. Run cold water over the pasta and set aside to cool.

For the tomato-kale chicken:

Heat the olive oil in a medium pot, season the chicken with salt, black pepper, and sear in the oil until golden brown on the outside. Transfer to a plate and set aside.

Add the onion and garlic to the oil and cook until softened and fragrant, 3 minutes.

Mix in the tomatoes and chicken broth, cover and cook over low heat until the tomatoes soften and the liquid reduces by half. Season with salt and black pepper.

Return the chicken to the pot and stir in the kale. Allow wilting for 2 minutes.

Divide the keto linguine onto serving plates, top with the kale sauce and then the Parmigianino-Reggiano cheese.

Garnish with the pine nuts and serve warm.

Nutrition:

Calories 740; Fats 52.9g; Carbs 15.1g; Net Carbs 6.1g; Protein 50.2g

131. Cajun Chicken Fettuccine

Preparation Time: 45 minutes + overnight chilling time
Servings: 4

Ingredients

For the keto fettuccine:

1 cup shredded mozzarella cheese

1 egg yolk

For the Cajun chicken:

2 tbsp olive oil

4 chicken breasts, cut into 1-inch cubes

1 medium yellow onion, thinly sliced

1 medium red bell pepper, deseeded and thinly sliced

1 medium green bell pepper, deseeded and thinly sliced

4 garlic cloves, minced

4 tsp Cajun seasoning

1 cup sugar-free Alfredo sauce

½ cup sugar-free marinara sauce

2 cups grated mozzarella cheese

½ cup grated Parmesan cheese

2 tbsp chopped fresh parsley

Directions

For the keto fettucine:

Pour the cheese into a medium safe-microwave bowl and melt in the microwave for 2 minutes while stirring at 20-second intervals until fully melted.

Take out the bowl and allow cooling for 1 minute only to warm the cheese but not cool completely. Mix in the egg yolk until well-combined.

Lay a parchment paper on a flat surface, pour the cheese mixture on top and cover with another parchment paper. Using a rolling pin, flatten the dough into 1/8-inch thickness.

Take off the parchment paper and cut the dough into thick fettuccine strands. Place in a bowl and refrigerate overnight. When ready to cook, bring

2 cups of water to a boil in medium saucepan and add the keto fettuccine. Cook for 40 seconds to 1 minute and then drain through a colander. Run cold water over the pasta and set aside to cool.

For the Cajun chicken:

Preheat the oven to 350 F and grease a baking dish with cooking spray.

Heat the olive oil in a medium skillet, season the chicken with salt, and black pepper, cook in the oil until seared on the outside, 6 minutes. Transfer to a plate.

Add the onion and bell peppers to the skillet and cook until softened, 5 minutes. Stir in the garlic and cook until fragrant, 30 seconds.

Return the chicken to the pot and stir in the Cajun seasoning, Alfredo sauce, and marinara sauce. Cook for 3 minutes over low heat.

Stir in the keto fettuccine until well-coated in the sauce and transfer the mixture to the baking dish.

Cover with the mozzarella and Parmesan cheeses, and bake in the oven until the cheeses melt and are golden brown on top, 15 minutes.

Remove from the oven, garnish with the parsley and serve warm.

Nutrition:

Calories 777; Fats 38.3g; Net Carbs 4.6g; Protein 92.8g

132.   Saffron Chicken And Pasta

Preparation Time: 35 minutes + overnight chilling time
Servings: 4

Ingredients

For the keto fettuccine:

1 cup shredded mozzarella cheese

1 egg yolk

For the saffron chicken:

3 tbsp butter

4 chicken breasts, cut into strips

½ tsp ground saffron threads

1 yellow onion, finely chopped

2 garlic cloves, minced

1 tbsp almond flour

1 pinch cardamom powder

1 pinch cinnamon powder

1 cup heavy cream

1 cup chicken stock

¼ cup chopped scallions

3 tbsp chopped parsley

Salt and black pepper to taste

Directions

For the keto fettuccine:

Pour the cheese into a medium safe-microwave bowl and melt in the microwave for 2 minutes while stirring at 20-second intervals until fully melted.

Take out the bowl and allow cooling for 1 minute only to warm the cheese but not cool completely. Mix in the egg yolk until well-combined.

Lay a parchment paper on a flat surface, pour the cheese mixture on top and cover with another parchment paper. Using a rolling pin, flatten the dough into 1/8-inch thickness.

Take off the parchment paper and cut the dough into thick fettuccine strands. Place in a bowl and refrigerate overnight.

When ready to cook, bring 2 cups of water to a boil in medium saucepan and add the keto fettuccine. Cook for 40 seconds to 1 minute and then drain through a colander. Run cold water over the pasta and set aside to cool.

For the saffron chicken:

Melt the butter in a large skillet, season the chicken with salt, black pepper, and cook in the oil until golden brown on the outside, 5 minutes.

Stir in the saffron, onion, garlic and cook until the onion softens and the garlic and saffron are fragrant, 3 minutes.

Stir in the almond flour, cardamom powder, cinnamon powder, and cook for 1 minute to exude some fragrance.

Add the heavy cream, chicken stock and cook for 2 to 3 minutes.

Adjust the taste with salt, black pepper and mix in the keto fettucine and scallions. Allow warming for 1 to 2 minutes and turn the heat off.

Dish the food onto serving plates and garnish with the parsley.

Serve warm.

Nutrition:

Calories 775; Fats 48.1g; Net Carbs 3.1g; Protein 73.4g

133. Mustard Chicken Shirataki

Preparation Time: 40 minutes
Servings: 4

Ingredients

For the shirataki angel hair:

2 (8 oz) packs angel hair shirataki

For the mustard chicken sauce:

1 tbsp olive oil

4 chicken breasts, cut into strips

Salt and black pepper to taste

1 yellow onion, finely sliced

1 yellow bell pepper, deseeded and sliced

1 garlic clove, minced

1 tbsp wholegrain mustard

5 tbsp heavy cream

1 cup chopped mustard greens

1 tbsp chopped parsley

Directions

For the shirataki angel hair:

Boil 2 cups of water in a medium pot over medium heat. Srain the shirataki pasta and rinse very well under hot running water. Allow proper draining and pour the shirataki pasta into the boiling water. Take off the heat and let sit for 3 minutes and strain again. Place a dry skillet over medium heat and stir-fry the shirataki pasta until visibly dry, and makes a squeaky sound when stirred, 1 to 2 minutes. Take off the heat and set aside.

For the mustard chicken sauce:

Heat the olive oil in a large skillet, season the chicken with salt, black pepper, and cook in the oil until golden brown, 10 minutes. Set aside. Stir in the onion, bell pepper and cook until softened, 5 minutes. Mix in the garlic and cook until fragrant, 30 seconds.

Mix in the mustard and heavy cream; simmer for 2 minutes and mix in the chicken and mustard greens. Allow wilting for 2 minutes and adjust the taste with salt and black pepper.

Stir in the shirataki pasta, allow warming for 1 minute and dish the food onto serving plates. Garnish with the parsley and serve warm.

Nutrition:

Calories 692; Fats 38.3g; Net Carbs 15.7g; Protein 64.8g

134.   Creamy Mushrooms With Broccoli Pasta

Preparation Time: 20 minutes
Servings: 4

Ingredients

4 large broccoli

2 tbsp olive oil

1 cup sliced cremini mushrooms

2 garlic cloves, minced

4 scallions, chopped

2 tbsp almond flour

1 ½ cups almond milk

2/3 cup grated Gruyere cheese

Salt and black pepper to taste

¼ cup chopped fresh parsley

Directions

Cut off the florets of the broccoli heads leaving only the stems. Cut the ends of the stem flatly and evenly. Run the stems through a spiralizer to make the noodles.

Heat the olive oil in a large skillet and sauté the broccoli noodles and mushrooms until softened, 5 to 7 minutes. Stir in the garlic and scallions; cook until fragrant, 1 minute.

In a medium bowl, combine the almond flour and almond milk, and pour the mixture over the vegetables. Stir and allow thickening for 2 to 3 minutes.

Whisk in half of the Gruyere cheese to melt and adjust the taste with salt and black pepper.

Dish the food onto serving plates, garnish with the remaining Gruyere cheese and parsley. Serve warm.

Nutrition:

Calories 221; Fats 15.6g; Net Carbs 1.41g; Protein 9.3g

135.   Cauliflower Casserole With Shirataki

Preparation Time: 45 minutes

Servings: 4

Ingredients

For the shirataki angel hair:

2 (8 oz) packs spinach angel hair shirataki

For the casserole:

1 medium head cauliflower, cut into florets

1 cup heavy cream

1 cup grated Monterey Jack cheese

1 tsp dried thyme

1 tsp smoked paprika

Salt to taste

½ tsp red chili flakes

Directions

For the shirataki angel hair:

Boil 2 cups of water in a medium pot over medium heat. Strain the shirataki pasta through a colander and rinse very well under hot running water. Allow proper draining and pour the shirataki pasta into the boiling water. Take off the heat and let sit for 3 minutes and strain again.

Place a dry skillet over medium heat and stir-fry the shirataki pasta until visibly dry, and makes a squeaky sound when stirred, 1 to 2 minutes. Take off the heat and set aside.

For the casserole:

Preheat the oven to 350 F and grease a baking dish with cooking spray. Set aside.

Bring 4 cups of water to a boil in a large pot and blanch the cauliflower for 4 minutes. Drain through a colander.

In a large bowl, mix the cauliflower, shirataki, heavy cream, half of the Monterey Jack cheese, thyme, paprika, salt, and red chili flakes until well-combined.

Transfer the mixture to the baking dish and top with the remaining cheese.

Bake for 30 minutes. Allow cooling for 2 minutes and serve afterwards.

Nutrition:

Calories 301; Fats 20.8g; Net Carbs 13.4g; Protein 11.6g

136.   Tofu Spaghetti Bolognese

Preparation Time: 25 minutes

Servings: 4

Ingredients

For the pasta:

2 tbsp butter

4 large parsnips, spiralized

Salt to taste

For the tofu Bolognese:

2 tbsp olive oil

1 cup pressed and crumbled firm tofu

1 medium white onion, chopped

2 celery stalks, finely chopped

1 garlic clove, minced

1 bay leaf

2 cups sugar-free passata

¼ cup vegetable broth

Salt and black pepper to taste

1 small bunch basil, chopped

1 cup grated Parmesan cheese for topping

Directions

For the pasta:

Melt the butter in a medium skillet and sauté the parsnips until tender, 5 to 7 minutes. Season with salt and set aside for serving.

For the tofu Bolognese:

Heat the olive oil in a large pot and cook the tofu until brown, 5 minutes.

Stir in the onion, celery, and cook until softened, 5 minutes. Add the garlic, bay leaf and cook until fragrant, 30 seconds.

Mix in the passata, vegetable broth and season with salt and black pepper. Cover the pot and cook until the sauce thickens, 8 to 10 minutes.

Open the lid, stir in the basil and adjust the taste with salt and black pepper.

Divide the pasta onto serving plates and top with the Bolognese.

Sprinkle the Parmesan cheese on top and serve warm.

Nutrition:

Calories 424; Fats 19.8g; Net Carbs 30.9g; Protein 21.7g

137. Balsamic Veggie-Pasta Mix

Preparation Time: 25 minutes + overnight chilling time
Servings: 4

Ingredients

For the keto penne:

1 cup shredded mozzarella cheese

1 egg yolk

For the balsamic mix:

3 tbsp olive oil

1 medium red onion, thinly sliced

1 lb green beans, trimmed and halved

1 head broccoli, cut into florets

1 red bell pepper, deseeded and thinly sliced

5 garlic cloves, minced

Salt and black pepper to taste

1 tsp dried oregano

3 tbsp organic balsamic vinegar

1 cup grated Parmigiano-Reggiano cheese

2 tbsp chopped walnuts for topping

Directions

For the keto penne:

Pour the cheese into a medium safe-microwave bowl and melt in the microwave for 2 minutes while stirring at 20-second intervals until fully melted.

Take out the bowl and allow cooling for 1 minute only to warm the cheese but not cool completely. Mix in the egg yolk until well-combined.

Lay a parchment paper on a flat surface, pour the cheese mixture on top and cover with another parchment paper. Using a rolling pin, flatten the dough into 1/8-inch thickness.

Take off the parchment paper and cut the dough into mimicked penne-size pieces. Place in a bowl and refrigerate overnight. When ready to cook, bring 2 cups of water to a boil in medium saucepan and add the keto penne. Cook for 40 seconds to 1 minute and then drain through a colander. Run cold water over the pasta and set aside to cool.

For the balsamic mix:

Heat the olive oil in a large skillet and sauté the onion, green beans, broccoli, and bell pepper until softened, 5 to 7 minutes.

Stir in the garlic and cook until fragrant, 30 seconds, and season with salt, black pepper, and oregano.

Mix in the balsamic vinegar, cook for 1 minute and toss in the keto penne. Allow warming for 1 minute.

Adjust the taste with salt, black pepper and spoon the food onto serving plates.

Garnish with the Parmigiano-Reggiano cheese and walnuts.

Serve warm.

Nutrition:

Calories 326; Fats 21.2g; Net Carbs 7.5g; Protein 20g

138.   Vegetarian Fajita Pasta

Preparation Time: 20 minutes + chilling time
Servings: 4

Ingredients

For the keto penne:

1 cup shredded mozzarella cheese

1 egg yolk

For the fajita mix:

1 tsp olive oil

6 garlic cloves, minced

2 cups sugar-free enchilada sauce

1 tsp cumin powder

½ tsp smoked paprika

1 tsp chili powder

1 cup chopped mixed bell peppers

Salt and black pepper to taste

For topping:

¾ cup chopped green onions

1 large avocado, pitted, peeled and sliced

Directions

For the keto penne:

Pour the cheese into a medium safe-microwave bowl and melt in the microwave for 2 minutes while stirring at 20-second intervals.Take out the bowl and allow cooling for 1 minute only to warm the cheese but not cool completely. Mix in the egg yolk.

Lay a parchment paper on a flat surface, pour the cheese mixture on top and cover with another parchment paper. Using a rolling pin, flatten the dough into 1/8-inch thickness.

Take off the parchment paper and cut the dough into penne shapes. Refrigerate overnight. Bring 2 cups of water to a boil in saucepan and add the penne. Cook for 1 minute and then drain through a colander. Run cold water over the pasta and set aside to cool.

For the fajita mix:

Heat olive oil in a skillet and sauté garlic for 30 seconds. Mix in enchilada sauce, cumin powder, paprika, chili powder, bell peppers, salt, and pepper. Cook for 5 minutes. Add penne and mix well. Top with the green onions and avocado.

Nutrition:

Calories 151; Fats 7.9g; Net Carbs 3.3g; Protein 11.9g

139.   Roasted Vegetable Spaghetti

Preparation Time: 45 minutes
Servings: 4

Ingredients

For the shirataki spaghetti:

2 (8 oz) packs shirataki spaghetti

Salt to season

For the roasted vegetable mix:

1 lb asparagus, trimmed and cut into ½ -inch pieces

1 cup broccoli florets

1 cup chopped mixed bell peppers

1 cup green beans, trimmed and halved

3 tbsp olive oil

Salt and black pepper to taste

1 small onion, chopped

2 garlic cloves, minced

1 cup diced tomatoes

½ cup grated Parmesan cheese for topping

½ cup chopped fresh basil for garnishing

Directions

For the shirataki spaghetti:

Boil 2 cups of water in a medium pot over medium heat. Strain the shirataki pasta through a colander and rinse very well under hot running water.Allow proper draining and pour the shirataki pasta into the boiling water. Cook for 3 minutes and strain again.

Place a dry skillet over medium heat and stir-fry the shirataki pasta until visibly dry, and makes a squeaky sound when stirred, 1 to 2 minutes. Take off the heat and set aside.

For the roasted vegetable mix:

Preheat the oven to 425 F.

In a bowl, add asparagus, broccoli, bell peppers, green beans and toss with half of the olive oil, some salt and black pepper. Spread the vegetables on a baking sheet and roast in the oven until tender and slightly charred, 20 minutes. Meanwhile, occasionally mix.

Heat the remaining olive oil in a skillet and sauté onion and garlic for 3 minutes. Stir in tomatoes and cook for 8 minutes. Mix in shirataki spaghetti and roasted vegetables. Top with the Parmesan cheese and basil. Serve warm.

Nutrition:

Calories 272; Fats 11.5g; Net Carbs 20.9g; Protein 12.1g

140. Spicy Veggie Pasta Bake

Preparation Time: 45 minutes + overnight chilling time
Servings: 4

Ingredients

For the keto penne:

1 cup shredded mozzarella cheese

1 egg yolk

For the veggie bake:

1 tbsp olive oil

1 cup mixed chopped bell peppers

1 yellow squash, chopped

1 red onion, halved and sliced

1 cup sliced white button mushrooms

Salt and black pepper to taste

¼ tsp red chili flakes

1 cup sugar-free marinara sauce

1 cup grated mozzarella cheese

1 cup grated Parmesan cheese

¼ cup chopped fresh basil

Directions

For the keto penne:

Pour the cheese into a medium safe-microwave bowl and melt in the microwave for 2 minutes while stirring at 20-second intervals until fully melted.

Take out the bowl and allow cooling for 1 minute only to warm the cheese but not cool completely. Mix in the egg yolk until well-combined.

Lay a parchment paper on a flat surface, pour the cheese mixture on top and cover with another parchment paper. Using a rolling pin, flatten the dough into 1/8-inch thickness.

Take off the parchment paper and cut the dough into penne-size pieces. Place in a bowl and refrigerate overnight. When ready to cook, bring 2 cups of water to a boil in medium saucepan and add the keto penne. Cook for 40 seconds to 1 minute and then drain through a colander. Run cold water over the pasta and set aside to cool.

For the veggie bake:

Heat the olive oil in a large cast iron and sauté the bell peppers, squash, onion, and mushrooms. Cook until softened, 5 minutes. Stir in the garlic and cook until fragrant, 30 seconds. Season with the salt, black pepper, and red chili flakes.

Mix in the marinara sauce and cook for 5 minutes.

Stir in the keto penne and spread the mozzarella and Parmesan cheeses on top.

Bake in the oven until the cheeses melt and golden brown on top, 15 minutes.

Remove from the oven, allow cooling for 2 minutes and dish onto serving plates.

Serve warm.

Nutrition:

Calories 248; Fats 11.5g; Net Carbs 4.9g; Protein 26.8g

141.   Super Green Pasta Skillet

Preparation Time: 15 minutes + overnight chilling time
Servings: 4

Ingredients

For the keto fettuccine:

1 cup shredded mozzarella cheese

1 egg yolk

For the green sauce:

2 garlic cloves, minced

1 lemon, juiced

1 cup baby spinach

½ cup almond milk

1 small avocado, pitted and peeled

1 tbsp olive oil

Salt to taste

1 cup grated Pecorino Romano cheese

Directions

For the keto fettuccine:

Pour the cheese into a medium safe-microwave bowl and melt in the microwave for 2 minutes while stirring at 20-second intervals until fully melted.

Take out the bowl and allow cooling for 1 minute only to warm the cheese but not cool completely. Mix in the egg yolk until well-combined.

Lay a parchment paper on a flat surface, pour the cheese mixture on top and cover with another parchment paper. Using a rolling pin, flatten the dough into 1/8-inch thickness.

Take off the parchment paper and cut the dough into thick fettuccine strands. Place in a bowl and refrigerate overnight.

When ready to cook, bring 2 cups of water to a boil in medium saucepan and add the keto fettucine. Cook for 40 seconds to 1 minute and then drain through a colander. Run cold water over the pasta and set aside to cool.

For the green sauce:

In a blender, combine the garlic, lemon juice, spinach, almond milk, avocado, olive oil, and salt. Process until smooth. Pour the keto fettucine into a medium bowl, top with the sauce and mix well. Top with the Pecorino Romano cheese and serve warm.

Nutrition:

Calories 290; Fats 19.2g; Net Carbs 5.3g; Protein 18.2g

142.   Broccoli And Pepper Spaghetti

Preparation Time: 20 minutes

Servings: 4

Ingredients

2 tbsp olive oil

4 zucchinis, spiralized

1 head broccoli, cut into florets

1 cup sliced mixed bell peppers

4 shallots, finely chopped

Salt and black pepper to taste

2 garlic cloves, minced

¼ tsp red pepper flakes

1 cup chopped kale

2 tbsp organic balsamic vinegar

½ lemon, juiced

1 cup grated Parmesan cheese

Directions

Heat the olive oil in a large skillet and sauté the turnips, broccoli, bell peppers, and shallots until softened, 7 minutes. Mix in the garlic, red pepper flakes and cook until fragrant, 30 seconds.

Stir in the kale and zucchinis; cook until tender, 2 to 3 minutes.

Mix in the vinegar, lemon juice and adjust the taste with salt and black pepper.

Dish the food onto serving plates and garnish with the Parmesan cheese.

Serve warm.

Nutrition:

Calories 199; Fats 13.9g; Net Carbs 5.9g; Protein 8.8g

143.   Veggie Pasta Primavera

Preparation Time: 25 minutes + overnight chilling time
Servings: 4

Ingredients

For the keto penne:

1 cup shredded mozzarella cheese

1 egg yolk

For the veggie mix:

¼ cup olive oil

½ cup chopped fresh green (spring) onions

2 cups cauliflower florets, cut into matchsticks

1 red bell pepper, deseeded and thinly sliced

4 garlic cloves, minced

1 cup grape tomatoes, halved

2 tsp dried Italian seasoning

½ lemon, juiced

½ cup grated Pecorino Romano cheese

2 tbsp chopped fresh parsley

Directions

For the keto penne:

Pour the cheese into a medium safe-microwave bowl and melt in the microwave for 2 minutes while stirring at 20-second intervals until fully melted.Take out the bowl and allow cooling for 1 minute only to warm the cheese but not cool completely. Mix in the egg yolk until well-combined.

Lay a parchment paper on a flat surface, pour the cheese mixture on top and cover with another parchment paper. Using a rolling pin, flatten the dough into 1/8-inch thickness. Take off the parchment paper and cut the dough into penne-size pieces. Place in a bowl and refrigerate overnight. Bring 2 cups of water to a boil in saucepan and add the keto penne. Cook for 1 minute and then drain. Set aside to cool.

For the veggie mix:

Heat olive oil in a skillet and sauté onion, cauliflower, and bell pepper for 7 minutes. Mix in garlic and cook until fragrant, 30 seconds. Stir in the tomatoes and Italian seasoning; cook until the tomatoes soften, 5 minutes. Mix in the lemon juice, keto penne and adjust the taste with salt and black pepper. Garnish with the Pecorino Romano cheese.

Nutrition:

Calories 283; Fats 18.5g; Net Carbs 5.2g; Protein 15.2g

144.   Vegan Lo Mein With Korean Tofu Bulgogi

Serving: 6
Preparation Time: 20 Minutes
Cooking Time: 45 Minutes

Ingredients

1 (14 ounce) package firm tofu

1 cup soy sauce

3 tablespoons sesame oil

2 tablespoons maple syrup

2 green onions, chopped

2 tablespoons Korean red pepper powder (optional)

1 tablespoon toasted sesame seeds

3 cloves minced garlic

1 teaspoon liquid smoke flavoring

7 ounces vegan lo mein noodles

1 tablespoon coconut oil

1 tablespoon sesame oil

1 onion, sliced

1 (10 ounce) package broccoli coleslaw mix

1/2 (8 ounce) package coleslaw mix

1 tablespoon coconut oil

salt and ground black pepper to taste

Direction

Preheat the oven to 375 degrees F (190 degrees C).

Place tofu onto a plate and place another plate on top. Set a 3- to 5-pound weight on top. Press tofu for 20 to 30 minutes; drain and discard the accumulated liquid. Dice into bite-sized cubes.

Combine soy sauce, 3 tablespoons sesame oil, maple syrup, green onions, red pepper powder, sesame seeds, garlic, and liquid smoke in a bowl. Fold in tofu and cover with plastic wrap. Place in the refrigerator to soak for no longer than 1 hour. Drain tofu, reserving marinade. Spread tofu evenly on a baking sheet.

Bake in the preheated oven until browned, 20 to 25 minutes.

Bring a large pot of lightly salted water to a boil. Cook lo mein noodles in boiling water, stirring occasionally, until noodles are tender yet firm to the bite, 10 to 12 minutes. Drain.

Combine coconut oil and 1 tablespoon sesame oil in a wok or saucepan over medium-high heat. Sauté onion until golden brown, about 2 minutes. Add broccoli coleslaw mix and coleslaw mix; sauté until wilted, about 3 minutes more. Reduce heat to medium-low; add cooked noodles, baked tofu, and reserved marinade. Simmer until heated through and all liquid is absorbed, about 5 minutes. Season with salt and pepper.

Nutrition:

Calories: 382 calories

Total Fat: 20.2 g

Cholesterol: 2 mg

Sodium: 2496 mg

Total Carbohydrate: 42.9 g

Protein: 13.2 g

145.   Vegan Mac And No Cheese

Serving: 4
Preparation Time: 15 Minutes
Cooking Time: 45 Minutes

Ingredients

1 (8 ounce) package uncooked elbow macaroni

1 tablespoon vegetable oil

1 medium onion, chopped

1 cup cashews

1/3 cup lemon juice

1 1/3 cups water

salt to taste

1/3 cup canola oil

4 ounces roasted red peppers, drained

3 tablespoons nutritional yeast

1 teaspoon garlic powder

1 teaspoon onion powder

Direction

Preheat oven to 350 degrees F (175 degrees C).

Bring a large pot of lightly salted water to a boil. Add macaroni, and cook for 8 to 10 minutes or until al dente; drain. Transfer to a medium baking dish.

Heat vegetable oil in a medium saucepan over medium heat. Stir in onion, and cook until tender and lightly browned. Gently mix with the macaroni.

In a blender or food processor, mix cashews, lemon juice, water, and salt. Gradually blend in canola oil, roasted red peppers, nutritional yeast, garlic powder, and onion powder. Blend until smooth. Thoroughly mix with the macaroni and onions.

Bake 45 minutes in the preheated oven, until lightly browned. Cool 10 to 15 minutes before serving.

Nutrition:

Calories: 648 calories

Total Fat: 39.2 g

Cholesterol: 0 mg

Sodium: 329 mg

Total Carbohydrate: 61.6 g

Protein: 16.5 g

146.   Vegan Portobello Stroganoff

Serving: 4
Preparation Time: 10 Minutes
Cooking Time: 40 Minutes

Ingredients

8 ounces vegan sour cream (such as Tofutti®)

1/2 cup water

3 tablespoons dried minced onion

2 tablespoons all-purpose flour

2 teaspoons vegan no-beef bouillon

1/4 teaspoon garlic powder

1/4 teaspoon dried basil

1/4 teaspoon ground black pepper

1/2 cup dry red wine

1 tablespoon olive oil

2 tablespoons soy sauce

1 tablespoon balsamic vinegar

2 cloves garlic, minced

2 large portobello mushroom caps, stems and gills removed

cooking spray

1/4 cup water, or as needed (optional)

Direction

Whisk vegan sour cream, 1/2 cup water, minced onion, flour, vegan bouillon, garlic powder, basil, and black pepper in a bowl. Cover and refrigerate.

Preheat oven to 400 degrees F (200 degrees C).

Whisk red wine, olive oil, soy sauce, balsamic vinegar, and garlic in another bowl.

Arrange mushroom caps with gill sides up in a baking dish and pour red wine mixture on top. Marinate for 20 minutes, then cover baking dish with aluminum foil.

Bake mushrooms in the preheated oven for 30 minutes. Remove foil, flip mushrooms, and continue baking until very tender, about 10 minutes more. Set aside to cool; dice mushrooms.

Heat a saucepan sprayed with cooking spray over medium heat. Cook and stir mushrooms in sauce pan until lightly browned, about 5 minutes; reduce heat to low.

Stir sour cream sauce into mushrooms. Continue to cook and stir until thickened, 1 to 2 minutes more. If the sauce becomes too thick, stir in 1/4 cup water.

Nutrition:

Calories: 259 calories

Total Fat: 13.5 g

Cholesterol: 0 mg

Sodium: 778 mg

Total Carbohydrate: 25.9 g

Protein: 3.3 g

147.   Vegan Pumpkin Macaroni And Cheese

Serving: 3
Preparation Time: 15 Minutes
Cooking Time: 15 Minutes

Ingredients

8 ounces penne pasta

2 tablespoons flour

1 tablespoon extra-virgin olive oil

1/2 cup oat milk

8 ounces pumpkin puree

2 teaspoons garlic salt

5 ounces shredded vegan Cheddar-style cheese, divided (such as Daiya®)

Direction

Bring a large pot of lightly salted water to a boil. Add penne and cook, stirring occasionally, until tender yet firm to the bite, about 11 minutes. Drain pasta and return to the pot.

Combine flour and oil in the same pot and mix until a smooth paste is formed. Add oat milk slowly. Incorporate pumpkin, whisking until thoroughly combined. Add garlic salt and 4 ounces vegan cheese. Mix until smooth.

Set an oven rack about 6 inches from the heat source and preheat the oven's broiler.

Fill 3 individual oval gratin casserole dishes with the pasta mixture. Top equally with remaining vegan cheese.

Broil in the preheated oven until cheese is melted, 1 to 3 minutes. Serve warm.

Nutrition:

Calories: 547 calories

Total Fat: 19 g

Cholesterol: 0 mg

Sodium: 2117 mg

Total Carbohydrate: 74.1 g

Protein: 16.5 g

148.   Vegan Stirfry Noodles

Serving: 2
Preparation Time: 20 Minutes
Cooking Time: 15 Minutes

Ingredients

1/2 (8 ounce) package dried soba noodles

1 tablespoon oil, or as needed

1/4 cup onion

2 cloves garlic, finely chopped

1 cup assorted mushrooms

1/4 cup chopped eggplant

6 leaves bok choy, chopped

2 tablespoons soy sauce

1 teaspoon teriyaki sauce

ground black pepper to taste

1 teaspoon sesame oil

1 green onion, finely chopped

Direction

Bring a large pot of lightly salted water to a boil. Cook soba in boiling water, stirring occasionally, until noodles are tender yet firm to the bite, 5 to 6 minutes. Drain.

Heat oil in a large skillet over medium heat. Add onion and garlic and stir-fry for 1 minute. Toss in mushrooms and eggplant; cook for 2 minutes more. Add cooked soba noodles, bok choy, soy sauce, teriyaki sauce, and pepper. Cook until bok choy is tender, about 2 minutes.

Sprinkle sesame oil and green onion over vegetables and serve.

Nutrition:

Calories: 326 calories

Total Fat: 10 g

Cholesterol: 0 mg

Sodium: 1500 mg

Total Carbohydrate: 53 g

Protein: 12.2 g

149.   Vegan Thai Mac N Cheese

Serving: 6
Preparation Time: 15 Minutes
Cooking Time: 25 Minutes

Ingredients

1 1/2 cups sunflower seeds

2 (14 ounce) cans coconut milk, divided

1/2 cup red curry paste, or more to taste, divided

1/2 cup chopped fresh cilantro, or more to taste, divided

2 limes, juiced, divided

1/2 teaspoon salt, plus more for seasoning

1 (8 ounce) package elbow macaroni

1 (8 ounce) package broccoli florets

1 pinch curry powder, or more to taste

3 tablespoons nutritional yeast

1 teaspoon white sugar

Direction

Preheat oven to 350 degrees F (175 degrees C).

Place sunflower seeds in a bowl and pour in enough water to cover; soak for about 10 minutes.

Mix 1 1/2 cans coconut milk, 1/4 cup curry paste, 1/4 cup cilantro, juice of 1 lime, and 1/2 teaspoon salt together in a saucepan; cook and stir over medium-low heat until curry sauce is thickened, about 5 minutes.

Bring a large pot of lightly salted water to a boil. Cook elbow macaroni in the boiling water, stirring occasionally until cooked through but firm to the bite, 8 minutes. Drain and mix pasta into curry sauce; cook and stir over low heat.

Place a steamer insert into a saucepan and fill with water to just below the bottom of the steamer. Bring water to a boil. Add broccoli, cover, and steam until tender, about 2 minutes. Season broccoli with salt and curry powder and transfer to a 9x13-inch baking dish.

Drain sunflower seeds and place in a blender with remaining coconut cream, remaining curry paste, remaining cilantro, juice of 1 lime, nutritional yeast, and sugar; blend until thick and smooth.

Spoon pasta mixture over broccoli. Pour sunflower seed mixture over pasta and stir to coat evenly.

Bake in the preheated oven until sauce is bubbling, about 10 minutes.

Nutrition:

Calories: 653 calories

Total Fat: 47.3 g

Cholesterol: 0 mg

Sodium: 613 mg

Total Carbohydrate: 47.3 g

Protein: 18.2 g

150.   Vegetable Cashew Saute

Serving: 8
Preparation Time: 30 Minutes
Cooking Time: 15 Minutes

Ingredients

1 (16 ounce) package whole wheat rotini pasta

2 tablespoons dark sesame oil

1/4 cup soy sauce

1/4 cup balsamic vinegar

2 tablespoons white sugar

1/4 cup dark sesame oil

3 cups chopped broccoli

1 cup chopped carrots

1 cup chopped red bell pepper

2 cups chopped fresh shiitake mushrooms

1 cup shelled edamame (green soybeans)

3/4 cup chopped unsalted cashew nuts

Direction

Bring a large pot of lightly salted water to a boil. Cook the rotini 10 to 12 minutes, until al dente, and drain.

In a small bowl, mix the 2 tablespoons sesame oil, soy sauce, vinegar, and sugar.

Heat the 1/4 cup sesame oil in a skillet over medium heat. Stir in the broccoli, carrots, red bell pepper, mushrooms, shelled edamame, and cashews. Mix in the sesame oil sauce. Cover skillet, and cook 5 minutes, or until vegetables are tender but crisp. Serve over the cooked pasta.

Nutrition:

Calories: 446 calories

Total Fat: 19.3 g

Cholesterol: 0 mg

Sodium: 494 mg

Total Carbohydrate: 57.2 g

Protein: 16.3 g

151. Vegetable Stuffed Cannelloni

Serving: 8
Preparation Time: 45 Minutes
Cooking Time: 1 h 5 Minutes

Ingredients

8 cannelloni noodles

5 cloves garlic, minced

5 shallots, chopped

2 tablespoons olive oil

1 cup dry sherry

2 cups heavy whipping cream

salt and pepper to taste

1 onion, chopped

1 cup fresh sliced mushrooms

1 zucchini, chopped

1 small eggplant, diced

2 roasted red bell peppers, diced

1 teaspoon dried basil

1 teaspoon dried oregano

3/4 cup ricotta cheese

1 cup grated Parmesan cheese

Direction

In a large pot of salted water, parboil cannelloni. (Parboiling is partially cooking the noodles in boiling water; they will finish cooking when baked.)

Meanwhile, cook 2 cloves garlic and 2 shallots in 1 tablespoon olive oil in a medium saucepan over medium heat for 30 seconds. Pour in sherry, raise heat to high, and reduce liquid by half. Stir in cream, and reduce until there is about 1 1/2 cups liquid. Remove from heat, and season with salt and pepper to taste. Set cream sauce aside.

In a large skillet, heat one tablespoon olive oil over medium heat. Cook onion, 3 shallots, 3 cloves garlic, mushrooms, zucchini, and eggplant in olive oil until all vegetables are tender. Transfer to a large bowl. Stir in red peppers, basil, oregano, ricotta, and Parmesan cheese. Season to taste with salt and pepper. Set filling aside.

Preheat oven to 350 degrees F (175 degrees C). Lightly grease one 9x13 inch baking dish. Stuff vegetable/cheese filling into cannelloni. Place in prepared baking dish, and cover with cream sauce.

Bake in preheated oven for 25 minutes.

Nutrition:

Calories: 424 calories

Total Fat: 28.9 g

Cholesterol: 90 mg

Sodium: 290 mg

Total Carbohydrate: 28.8 g

Protein: 10 g

152.   Aunty Pastos Seafood Lasagna

Serving: 8
Preparation Time: 5 Minutes
Cooking Time: 1 h 15 Minutes

Ingredients

8 lasagna noodles

2 tablespoons butter

1 cup chopped onion

1 (8 ounce) package cream cheese, softened

1 1/2 cups cottage cheese, creamed

1 egg, beaten

2 teaspoons dried basil

1/2 teaspoon salt

1/8 teaspoon ground black pepper

2 (10.75 ounce) cans condensed cream of mushroom soup

1/3 cup milk

1/3 cup dry white wine

1 (6 ounce) can crabmeat

1 pound cooked salad shrimp

1/4 cup grated Parmesan cheese

1/2 cup shredded sharp Cheddar cheese

2 cups fresh sliced mushrooms

Direction

Cook noodles in a large pot of boiling salted water until done. Rinse and drain noodles. Set aside.

Melt butter or margarine in a small sauté pan over medium heat. Add onion; cook and stir until tender. Add cream cheese, cottage cheese, egg, basil, and salt and pepper.

In a medium bowl, combine soup, milk, and wine. Stir in crab, shrimp, and mushrooms.

Place 4 noodles in the bottom of a well-oiled 9x13 inch pan. Spread 1/2 cheese mixture over the noodles, and spoon 1/2 soup mixture over cheese. Repeat layers.

Bake, uncovered, at 350 degrees F (175 degrees C) for 45 minutes. Top with sharp cheese, and parmesan cheese. Brown lasagna under broiler. Remove from oven, and let stand 15 minutes before serving.

Nutrition:

Calories: 475 calories

Total Fat: 25 g

Cholesterol: 209 mg

Sodium: 1217 mg

Total Carbohydrate: 28.2 g

Protein: 33.1 g

153.   Bacon N Egg Lasagna

Serving: 12
Preparation Time: 45 Minutes
Cooking Time: 35 Minutes

Ingredients

1 pound bacon strips, diced

1 large onion, chopped

1/3 cup all-purpose flour

1/2 to 1 teaspoon salt

1/4 teaspoon pepper

4 cups 2% milk

12 lasagna noodles, cooked and drained

12 hard-boiled large eggs, sliced

2 cups shredded Swiss cheese

1/3 cup grated Parmesan cheese

2 tablespoons minced fresh parsley, optional

Direction

In a large skillet, cook bacon until crisp. Remove with a slotted spoon to paper towels. Drain, reserving 1/3 cup drippings. In the drippings, sauté onion until tender. Stir in the flour, salt and pepper until blended. Gradually stir in milk. Bring to a boil; cook and stir for 2 minutes or until thickened. Remove from the heat. Spread 1/2 cup sauce in a greased 13-in. x 9-in. baking dish. Layer with four noodles, a third of the eggs and bacon, Swiss cheese and white sauce. Repeat layers twice. Sprinkle with Parmesan cheese. Bake, uncovered, at 350 degrees for 35-40 minutes or until bubbly. If desired, sprinkle with parsley. Let stand for 15 minutes before cutting.

Nutrition:

Calories: 386 calories

Total Fat: 20g

Cholesterol: 252mg

Sodium: 489mg

Total Carbohydrate: 28g

Protein: 23g

Fiber: 1g

154. Baked Lasagna Roll Ups

Serving: 4
Preparation Time: 20 Minutes
Cooking Time: 40 Minutes

Ingredients

1 package (10 ounces) frozen spinach, thawed and squeezed dry

1 large egg, beaten

1-3/4 cups ricotta cheese

4 tablespoons grated Parmesan cheese, divided

1/2 teaspoon salt

1/4 teaspoon pepper

1/8 teaspoon ground nutmeg

8 thin slices deli ham, halved lengthwise

8 lasagna noodles, cooked and drained

1 jar (14 ounces) spaghetti sauce

Direction

In a bowl, combine the spinach, egg, ricotta cheese, 2 tablespoons
Parmesan cheese, salt, pepper and nutmeg. Place two pieces of ham on
each noodle. Spread with 1/3 cup spinach mixture. Roll up and place seam
side down in a greased 13-in. x 9-in. baking dish. Top with spaghetti sauce.
Cover and bake at 350 degrees for 40-45 minutes or until heated through.
Uncover; sprinkle with remaining Parmesan. Let stand for 15 minutes before
cutting.

Nutrition:

Calories: 710 calories

Total Fat: 31g

Cholesterol: 181mg

Sodium: 3047mg

Total Carbohydrate: 57g

Protein: 53g

Fiber: 5g

155. Baked Mexican Lasagna

Serving: 6-8
Preparation Time: 20 Minutes
Cooking Time: 30 Minutes

Ingredients

1-1/2 pounds ground beef

1-1/2 teaspoons ground cumin

1 tablespoon chili powder

1/4 teaspoon garlic powder

1/4 teaspoon cayenne pepper

1 teaspoon salt or to taste

1 teaspoon pepper or to taste

1 can (14-1/2 ounces) diced tomatoes, drained

10 to 12 corn tortillas

2 cups (16 ounces) small curd 4% cottage cheese, drained

1 cup shredded pepper jack cheese

1 large egg

1/2 cup shredded cheddar cheese

2 cups shredded lettuce

1/2 cup chopped tomatoes

3 green onions, chopped

1/4 cup sliced ripe olives

Direction

In a large skillet, cook beef over medium heat until no longer pink; drain. Add the cumin, chili powder, garlic powder, cayenne, salt, pepper and tomatoes; heat through. Cover bottom and sides of a greased 13x9-in. baking dish with tortillas. Pour beef mixture over tortillas; place a layer of tortillas over meat mixture and set aside. Combine cottage cheese, Monterey Jack cheese and egg; pour over tortillas. Bake at 350 degrees for 30 minutes. Remove from oven; sprinkle rows of cheddar cheese, lettuce, tomatoes, green onions and olives diagonally across center of casserole.

Nutrition:

Calories: 381 calories

Total Fat: 19g

Cholesterol: 101mg

Sodium: 785mg

Total Carbohydrate: 23g

Protein: 30g

Fiber: 4g

156.   Beef And Spinach Lasagna

Serving: 12
Preparation Time: 40 Minutes
Cooking Time: 40 Minutes

Ingredients

1 pound lean ground beef (90% lean)

1 medium onion, chopped

2 jars (24 ounces each) spaghetti sauce

4 garlic cloves, minced

1 teaspoon dried basil

1 teaspoon dried oregano

1 package (10 ounces) frozen chopped spinach, thawed and squeezed dry

2 cups ricotta cheese

2 cups shredded part-skim mozzarella cheese, divided

9 no-cook lasagna noodles

Direction

In a large skillet, cook beef and onion over medium heat until meat is no longer pink; drain. Stir in the spaghetti sauce, garlic, basil and oregano. Bring to a boil. Reduce heat; cover and simmer for 10 minutes. In a large bowl, combine the spinach, ricotta and 1 cup mozzarella cheese. Spread 1-1/2 cups meat sauce into a greased 13x9-in. baking dish. Top with three noodles. Spread 1-1/2 cups sauce to edges of noodles. Top with half of the spinach mixture. Repeat layers. Top with the remaining noodles, sauce and mozzarella cheese. Cover and bake at 375 degrees for 30 minutes. Uncover; bake 10-15 minutes longer or until bubbly. Let stand for 10 minutes before cutting.

Nutrition:

Calories: 281 calories

Total Fat: 11g

Cholesterol: 50mg

Sodium: 702mg

Total Carbohydrate: 26g

Protein: 20g

Fiber: 3g

157.   Beef Enchilada Lasagna Casserole

Serving: 12
Preparation Time: 45 Minutes
Cooking Time: 30 Minutes

Ingredients

1-1/2 pounds ground beef

1 medium onion, chopped

1 garlic clove, minced

1 can (14-1/2 ounces) stewed tomatoes, undrained

1 can (10 ounces) enchilada sauce

1 to 2 teaspoons ground cumin

1 large egg, beaten

1-1/2 cups 4% cottage cheese

3 cups shredded Mexican cheese blend

8 flour tortillas (8 inches), cut in half

1 cup shredded cheddar cheese

Direction

In a large skillet, cook the beef, onion and garlic over medium heat until meat is no longer pink; drain. Stir in the tomatoes, enchilada sauce and cumin. Bring to a boil. Reduce heat; simmer, uncovered, for 20 minutes. In a small bowl, combine egg and cottage cheese; set aside. Spread a third of the meat sauce into a greased 13x9-in. baking dish. Layer with half of the tortillas, cottage cheese mixture, cheese blend and a third of the meat sauce. Repeat layers. Sprinkle with cheddar cheese. Cover and bake at 350 degrees for 20 minutes. Uncover; bake 10 minutes longer or until bubbly. Let stand for 15 minutes before cutting.

Nutrition:

Calories: 387 calories

Total Fat: 21g

Cholesterol: 87mg

Sodium: 771mg

Total Carbohydrate: 25g

Protein: 25g

Fiber: 1g

158.   Beef Lasagne

Serving: 12
Preparation Time: 40 Minutes
Cooking Time: 45 Minutes

Ingredients
1 pound ground beef
2 garlic cloves, minced
1-1/2 cups water
1 can (15 ounces) tomato sauce
1 can (6 ounces) tomato paste
1/2 to 1 envelope onion soup mix
1 teaspoon dried oregano
1/2 teaspoon sugar
1/4 teaspoon pepper
9 lasagna noodles, cooked and drained
2 cups 4% cottage cheese
4 cups shredded part-skim mozzarella cheese
2 cups grated Parmesan cheese
Direction
In a large saucepan, cook beef over medium heat until meat is no longer
pink. Add garlic; cook 1 minute longer. Drain. Stir in the water, tomato
sauce and paste, soup mix, oregano, sugar and pepper. Bring to a boil.
Reduce heat; cover and simmer for 30 minutes. Spoon 1/2 cup meat sauce
into a greased 13x9-in. baking dish. Layer with three noodles and a third of
the cottage cheese, mozzarella, meat sauce and Parmesan cheese. Repeat
layers twice. Cover and bake at 350 degrees for 40 minutes or until bubbly
and heated through. Uncover; bake 5-10 minutes longer. Let stand for 10
minutes before cutting.
Nutrition:
Calories: 367 calories
Total Fat: 18g
Cholesterol: 62mg
Sodium: 901mg
Total Carbohydrate: 25g
Protein: 27g
Fiber: 2g

159.   Black Bean Chicken Enchilada Lasagna

Serving: 8
Preparation Time: 30 Minutes
Cooking Time: 25 Minutes

Ingredients

2 cans (10 ounces each) enchilada sauce

12 corn tortillas (6 inches)

2 cups coarsely shredded rotisserie chicken

1 small onion, chopped

1 can (15 ounces) black beans, rinsed and drained

3 cans (4 ounces each) whole green chilies, drained and coarsely chopped

3 cups crumbled queso fresco or shredded Mexican cheese blend

2 medium ripe avocados

2 tablespoons sour cream

2 tablespoons lime juice

1/2 teaspoon salt

Chopped fresh tomatoes and cilantro

Direction

Preheat oven to 350 degrees. Spread 1/2 cup enchilada sauce into a greased 13x9-in. baking dish; top with four tortillas, 1 cup chicken, 1/4 cup onion, 1/4 cup beans, 1/3 cup green chilies and 1 cup cheese. Repeat layers. Drizzle with 1/2 cup enchilada sauce; top with the remaining tortillas, onion, beans, chilies, sauce and cheese. Bake, uncovered, 25-30 minutes or until bubbly and cheese is melted. Let stand 10 minutes before serving. Meanwhile, quarter, peel and pit one avocado; place avocado in a food processor. Add sour cream, lime juice and salt; process until smooth. Peel, pit and cut remaining avocado into small cubes. Top lasagna with tomatoes, cilantro and cubed avocado. Serve with avocado sauce.

Nutrition:

Calories: 407 calories

Total Fat: 18g

Cholesterol: 64mg

Sodium: 857mg

Total Carbohydrate: 39g

Protein: 28g

Fiber: 8g

160.　Black Bean Lasagna

Serving: 8
Preparation Time: 30 Minutes
Cooking Time: 35 Minutes

Ingredients

1 tablespoon vegetable oil

2 onions, chopped

4 cloves garlic, chopped

1/2 green bell pepper, diced

1/2 red bell pepper, diced

1 (14.5 ounce) can chopped tomatoes

1 cup salsa

2 (15 ounce) cans black beans, drained and rinsed

salt and black pepper to taste

2 avocados - peeled, pitted, and mashed

1 tablespoon fresh lemon juice

12 (6 inch) corn tortillas, quartered

2 cups shredded Cheddar cheese

Direction

Preheat oven to 400 degrees F (200 degrees C). Lightly grease a 9x13-inch baking dish.

Warm oil in a large skillet over medium heat. Stir in onions, 3 cloves of chopped garlic, and green and red bell peppers. Cook until the onions are soft and translucent. Stir in tomatoes with juice, salsa, and black beans. Season with salt and pepper. Bring to a simmer, and cook about 3 minutes.

In a bowl, mash the avocados with 1 clove chopped garlic and lemon juice.

Place a layer of tortillas on the bottom of the baking dish. Spread 1/3 of the tomato and bean mixture on top. Spread 1/2 of guacamole on top, then sprinkle with 1/3 of cheese. Lay out another layer of tortillas. Top with half of the remaining tomato and bean mixture. Then spread remaining guacamole on top. Sprinkle with half the cheese. Repeat with remaining ingredients.

Bake in preheated oven for 35 minutes, or until sauce is bubbly.

Nutrition:

Calories: 331 calories

Total Fat: 19.7 g

Cholesterol: 30 mg

Sodium: 472 mg

Total Carbohydrate: 29.8 g

Protein: 11.7 g

161.   Blue Cheese Lasagna

Serving: 8
Preparation Time: 30 Minutes
Cooking Time: 1 h 35 Minutes

Ingredients

cooking spray

Sauce:

1/2 pound ground beef

1/2 pound lean ground pork

1 (24 ounce) jar spaghetti sauce

2 tablespoons brown sugar

Cheese Layer:

1 cup cottage cheese

1 cup crumbled blue cheese

1/4 cup freshly grated Parmesan cheese

1 large egg, lightly beaten

1 tablespoon dried oregano

1 (12 ounce) box no-boil lasagna noodles

6 slices provolone cheese

1 cup shredded Cheddar cheese

Direction

Preheat oven to 300 degrees F (150 degrees C). Coat the inside of a glass 9x5-inch loaf pan with cooking spray. Line a baking sheet with aluminum foil.

Heat a large skillet over medium-high heat. Cook and stir beef and pork in the hot skillet until browned and crumbly, 5 to 7 minutes; drain and discard grease. Mix spaghetti sauce and brown sugar into beef-pork mixture until sauce is well blended.

Combine cottage cheese, blue cheese, Parmesan cheese, egg, and oregano in a bowl.

Spread enough sauce into the bottom of the loaf pan to reach 1-inch depth. Break 2 lasagna noodles to fit the length of the loaf pan, slightly overlapping. Spread 1/2 of the cheese mixture over noodle layer. Layer 3 slices provolone, slightly overlapping, over cheese layer. Sprinkle 1/2 of the Cheddar cheese over provolone cheese. Repeat layering with the remaining ingredients ending in a layer of sauce.

Place the loaf pan on the prepared baking sheet and top loaf pan loosely with a piece of aluminum foil.

Bake in the preheated oven until bubbling and cooked through, about 1 1/2 hours. Let stand for 15 minutes before slicing.

Nutrition:

Calories: 601 calories

Total Fat: 34.8 g

Cholesterol: 128 mg

Sodium: 1153 mg

Total Carbohydrate: 34.9 g

Protein: 36.5 g

162.   Brendas Lasagna

Serving: 8
Preparation Time: 30 Minutes
Cooking Time: 30 Minutes

Ingredients

1 (16 ounce) package lasagna noodles

1 pound lean ground beef

salt and pepper to taste

1 (16 ounce) jar spaghetti sauce

1 clove garlic, minced

1/2 pound shredded mozzarella cheese

1/2 pound shredded Cheddar cheese

1 pint ricotta cheese

Direction

Bring a large pot of lightly salted water to a boil. Add pasta and cook for 8 to 10 minutes or until al dente; drain.

Preheat oven to 350 degrees F (175 degrees C). In a large skillet over medium-high heat, brown beef and season with salt and pepper; drain. Stir in spaghetti sauce and garlic and simmer 5 minutes.

In a medium bowl, combine mozzarella, Cheddar and ricotta; stir well. In 9x13 inch pan, alternate layers of noodles, meat mixture and cheese mixture until pan is filled.

Bake in preheated oven for 30 minutes, or until cheese is melted and bubbly.

Nutrition:

Calories: 643 calories

Total Fat: 29.3 g

Cholesterol: 108 mg

Sodium: 707 mg

Total Carbohydrate: 53.4 g

Protein: 41.3 g

163.   Broccoli Chicken Lasagna

Serving: 12
Preparation Time: 20 Minutes
Cooking Time: 50 Minutes

Ingredients

1/2 pound sliced fresh mushrooms

1 large onion, chopped

1/4 cup butter, cubed

1/2 cup all-purpose flour

1/2 teaspoon salt

1/4 teaspoon pepper

1/8 teaspoon ground nutmeg

1 can (14-1/2 ounces) chicken broth

1-3/4 cups whole milk

2/3 cup grated Parmesan cheese

1 package (16 ounces) frozen broccoli cuts, thawed

9 lasagna noodles, cooked and drained

1-1/3 cups julienned fully cooked ham, divided

2 cups shredded Monterey Jack cheese, divided

2 cups cubed cooked chicken

Direction

Preheat oven to 350 degrees. In a large skillet, sauté mushrooms and onion in butter until tender. Stir in flour, salt, pepper and nutmeg until blended. Gradually stir in broth and milk. Bring to a boil; cook and stir 2 minutes or until thickened. Stir in Parmesan cheese and broccoli; heat through. Spread 1/2 cup broccoli mixture in a greased 13x9-in. baking dish. Layer with three noodles, a third of the remaining broccoli mixture, 1 cup ham and 1 cup Monterey Jack cheese. Top with three noodles, half the remaining broccoli mixture, all the chicken and 1/2 cup Monterey Jack cheese. Top with remaining noodles, broccoli mixture and ham. Cover and bake 45-50 minutes or until bubbly. Sprinkle with remaining Monterey Jack cheese. Bake 5 minutes longer or until cheese is melted. Let stand 15 minutes before cutting.

Nutrition:

Calories: 326 calories

Total Fat: 16g

Cholesterol: 64mg

Sodium: 703mg

Total Carbohydrate: 24g

Protein: 22g

Fiber: 2g

164.   Broccoli Lasagna

Serving: 6
Preparation Time: 20 Minutes
Cooking Time: 40 Minutes

Ingredients

9 lasagna noodles

3 tablespoons butter

1 small onion, chopped

2 cloves garlic, chopped

2 tablespoons all-purpose flour

1/4 teaspoon ground white pepper

1 teaspoon salt, divided

1/8 teaspoon ground nutmeg

2 1/2 cups milk

2 tablespoons chopped fresh parsley

1 (15 ounce) container ricotta cheese

1 (10 ounce) package chopped frozen broccoli, thawed and drained

1/4 cup grated Parmesan cheese

2 cups shredded mozzarella cheese, divided

Direction

Preheat oven to 350 degrees F (175 degrees C).

Bring a large pot of lightly salted water to a boil. Add pasta and cook for 8 to 10 minutes or until al dente; drain.

In a medium saucepan over medium heat, melt butter. Cook onion and garlic in butter until tender. Stir in flour, pepper, 1/2 teaspoon salt and nutmeg. Stirring continuously, pour in milk, a little at a time, allowing mixture to thicken. Bring to a boil for 1 minute, then remove from heat and stir in parsley. Set aside.

In a medium bowl, combine ricotta, broccoli, Parmesan, 1 cup of mozzarella and remaining 1/2 teaspoon salt. Stir until well blended.

In a 7x11 inch baking dish layer: 1/4 cup white sauce; 3 noodles; one-third of remaining white sauce; half the broccoli mixture; 3 more noodles; half remaining white sauce; remaining broccoli mixture; 3 noodles; remaining white sauce. Sprinkle with remaining mozzarella. Cover with foil coated with cooking spray.

Bake in preheated oven 30 minutes. Let stand 10 minutes before serving.

Nutrition:

Calories: 468 calories

Total Fat: 21.4 g

Cholesterol: 72 mg

Sodium: 858 mg

Total Carbohydrate: 41.7 g

Protein: 28.6 g

165.   Cheese Lovers Lasagna

Serving: 10
Preparation Time: 30 Minutes
Cooking Time: 25 Minutes

Ingredients

1 (16 ounce) package lasagna noodles

1 (16 ounce) jar spaghetti sauce with meat

1 (8 ounce) package mozzarella cheese, shredded

6 slices processed American cheese

1 (8 ounce) package mild Cheddar cheese, shredded

1 (8 ounce) container small curd cottage cheese

1/4 cup grated Parmesan cheese

Direction

Preheat oven to 350 degrees F (175 degrees C).

Bring a large pot of lightly salted water to a boil. Add lasagna pasta and cook for 8 to 10 minutes or until al dente; drain and rinse with cold water.

Line the bottom of a 9x13 inch casserole dish with noodles and spread on 1/4 cup of the spaghetti sauce. Add another layer of noodles and begin alternating layers of cheeses, noodles and sauce, beginning with the cottage cheese. Make sure you leave enough spaghetti sauce to cover the top to prevent hardening of the top layer of noodles. Finish with a sprinkle of Parmesan.

Bake in a preheated oven until cheese is well melted and filling is heated through; about 20 or 25 minutes.

Nutrition:

Calories: 448 calories

Total Fat: 20.6 g

Cholesterol: 61 mg

Sodium: 851 mg

Total Carbohydrate: 41 g

Protein: 25 g

166.   Cheesy Shell Lasagna

Serving: 12
Preparation Time: 25 Minutes
Cooking Time: 45 Minutes

Ingredients

1-1/2 pounds lean ground beef (90% lean)

2 medium onions, chopped

1 garlic clove, minced

1 can (14-1/2 ounces) diced tomatoes, undrained

1 jar (14 ounces) meatless spaghetti sauce

1 can (4 ounces) mushroom stems and pieces, undrained

8 ounces uncooked small shell pasta

2 cups (16 ounces) reduced-fat sour cream

11 slices (8 ounces) reduced-fat provolone cheese

1 cup shredded part-skim mozzarella cheese

Direction

In a nonstick skillet, cook beef and onions over medium heat until meat is no longer pink. Add garlic; cook 1 minute longer. Drain. Stir in the tomatoes, spaghetti sauce and mushrooms. Bring to a boil. Reduce heat; simmer, uncovered, for 20 minutes. Meanwhile, cook pasta according to package directions; drain. Place half of the pasta in an ungreased 13x9-in. baking dish. Top with half of the meat sauce, sour cream and provolone cheese. Repeat layers. Sprinkle with mozzarella cheese. Cover and bake at 350 degrees for 35-40 minutes. Uncover; bake 10 minutes longer or until the cheese begins to brown. Let stand for 10 minutes before cutting.

Nutrition:

Calories: 346 calories

Total Fat: 15g

Cholesterol: 50mg

Sodium: 515mg

Total Carbohydrate: 29g

Protein: 27g

Fiber: 2g

167.   Cheesy Tuna Lasagna

Serving: 6-8
Preparation Time: 15 Minutes
Cooking Time: 25 Minutes

Ingredients

1 medium onion, chopped

2 tablespoons butter

1 can (12 ounces) tuna, drained and flaked

1 can (10-3/4 ounces) condensed cream of mushroom soup, undiluted

1/2 cup 2% milk

1/2 teaspoon garlic salt

1/2 teaspoon dried oregano

1/4 teaspoon pepper

9 lasagna noodles, cooked and drained

1-1/2 cups (12 ounces) 4% cottage cheese

8 ounces sliced part-skim mozzarella cheese

1/4 cup grated Parmesan cheese

Direction

In a large saucepan, sauté onion in butter until tender. Stir in the tuna, soup, milk, garlic salt, oregano and pepper until combined. Spread 3/4 cupful into a greased 11x7-in. baking dish. Layer with three noodles (trimming if necessary), 3/4 cup tuna mixture, half of the cottage cheese and a third of the mozzarella cheese. Repeat layers. Top with remaining noodles, tuna mixture and mozzarella cheese. Sprinkle with Parmesan cheese. Bake, uncovered, at 350 degrees for 25-30 minutes or until bubbly. Let stand for 10-15 minutes before serving.

Nutrition:

Calories: 361 calories

Total Fat: 13g

Cholesterol: 51mg

Sodium: 909mg

Total Carbohydrate: 29g

Protein: 30g

Fiber: 2g

168.   Chicken Artichoke Lasagna

Serving: 8
Preparation Time: 30 Minutes
Cooking Time: 03 h 00 Minutes

Ingredients

2 cans (14 ounces each) water-packed artichoke hearts, drained and finely chopped

1 cup shredded Parmesan cheese, divided

1/4 cup loosely packed basil leaves, finely chopped

3 garlic cloves, minced, divided

1 pound ground chicken

1 tablespoon canola oil

1 cup finely chopped onion

3/4 teaspoon salt

1/2 teaspoon pepper

1/2 cup white wine

1 cup half-and-half cream

1 package (8 ounces) cream cheese, softened

1 cup shredded Monterey Jack cheese

1 large Nellie's Free Range Egg

1-1/2 cups (12 ounces) 2% cottage cheese

9 no-cook lasagna noodles

2 cups shredded part-skim mozzarella cheese

Prepared pesto, optional

Additional basil, optional

Direction

Fold two 18-in. square pieces of foil into thirds. Crisscross strips and place strips on bottom and up sides of a 6-qt. slow cooker. Coat strips with cooking spray. Combine artichoke hearts, 1/2 cup Parmesan cheese, basil and 2 garlic cloves. In a large skillet, crumble chicken over medium heat 6-8 minutes or until no longer pink; drain. Set chicken aside. Add oil and onion;

cook and stir just until tender, 6-8 minutes. Add salt, pepper and remaining garlic; cook 1 minute longer. Stir in wine. Bring to a boil; cook until liquid is reduced by half, 4-5 minutes. Stir in cream, cream cheese and Monterey Jack cheese. Return chicken to pan. In a bowl, combine egg, cottage cheese and remaining Parmesan. Spread 3/4 cup meat mixture into slow cooker. Layer with 3 noodles (breaking noodles as necessary to fit), 3/4 cup meat mixture, 1/2 cup cottage cheese mixture, 1 cup artichoke mixture and 1/2 cup mozzarella cheese. Repeat layers twice; top with remaining mozzarella cheese. Cook, covered, on low until noodles are tender, 3-4 hours. Remove slow cooker insert and let stand 30 minutes. If desired, serve with pesto and sprinkle with additional basil.

Nutrition:

Calories: 588 calories

Total Fat: 34g

Cholesterol: 144mg

Sodium: 1187mg

Total Carbohydrate: 31g

Protein: 36g

Fiber: 1g

169.   Chicken Alfredo Lasagna

Serving: 9
Preparation Time: 30 Minutes
Cooking Time: 1 h 10 Minutes

Ingredients

2 tablespoons olive oil

1 teaspoon dried oregano

1 teaspoon dried basil

2 boneless chicken breasts, diced

2 (14.5 ounce) cans diced tomatoes

2 (16 ounce) jars Alfredo sauce

1 (8 ounce) package oven-ready lasagna noodles

1 (8 ounce) container ricotta cheese, or as needed

1 (8 ounce) package shredded mozzarella cheese

1 (8 ounce) package shredded Parmesan cheese

Direction

Preheat oven to 350 degrees F (175 degrees C).

Heat olive oil, oregano, and basil in a skillet over medium-high heat; sauté chicken in hot oil until cooked through, about 10 minutes.

Mix tomatoes and Alfredo sauce together in a bowl.

Spread 1/3 of the sauce mixture in the bottom of a 9x13-inch baking dish; add 1/3 of the lasagna noodles. Spread 1/3 of the ricotta cheese over noodles and top with 1/4 of the mozzarella cheese and 1/4 of the Parmesan cheese. Repeat 1 more layer of 1/3 of the sauce mixture, 1/3 of the noodles, 1/3 of the ricotta cheese, 1/4 of the mozzarella cheese, and 1/3 of the Parmesan cheese. Spread chicken mixture over cheese layer and top with remaining 1/3 of the sauce mixture, 1/3 of the noodles, 1/3 of the ricotta cheese, 1/4 of the mozzarella cheese, and 1/4 of the Parmesan cheese. Cover dish with aluminum foil.

Bake in the preheated oven for 1 hour. Remove foil and sprinkle remaining 1/4 of the mozzarella cheese and 1/4 of the Parmesan cheese. Continue baking until cheeses are melted and lightly browned, about 15 minutes more.

Nutrition:

Calories: 629 calories

Total Fat: 46.8 g

Cholesterol: 102 mg

Sodium: 1706 mg

Total Carbohydrate: 21.4 g

Protein: 31.5 g

170.   Chicken And Broccoli Lasagna Rolls

Serving: 2 casseroles (3each).
Preparation Time: 20 Minutes
Cooking Time: 45 Minutes

Ingredients

1 small onion, chopped

3 tablespoons butter

3 tablespoons all-purpose flour

1 can (14-1/2 ounces) chicken broth

1 cup whole milk

1-1/2 cups shredded Monterey Jack cheese

3 cups diced cooked chicken

6 cups frozen chopped broccoli, thawed and drained

2 large eggs, lightly beaten

3/4 cup dry bread crumbs

1 jar (6-1/2 ounces) diced pimientos, drained

1/4 cup minced fresh parsley

1/2 teaspoon salt, optional

12 lasagna noodles, cooked and drained

Direction

In a large saucepan, sauté onion in butter until tender. Stir in flour until blended. Gradually add broth and milk. Bring to a boil; cook and stir for 2 minutes or until thickened. Remove from the heat; stir in cheese. Pour 1/3 cup each into two greased 8-in. square baking dishes; set aside. In a large bowl, combine 1 cup cheese sauce, chicken, broccoli, eggs, bread crumbs, pimientos, parsley and salt if desired. Spread about 1/2 cup over each noodle. Roll up jelly-roll style, beginning with a short side; secure ends with toothpicks. Place six roll-ups curly end down in each baking dish. Top with remaining cheese sauce. Cover and freeze one casserole for up to 3 months. Cover and bake second casserole at 350 degrees for 40 minutes or until a thermometer reads 160 degrees. Uncover; bake 5 minutes longer or until bubbly. Discard toothpicks. To use frozen casserole: Thaw in the refrigerator for 8 hours or overnight. Bake as directed.

Nutrition:

Calories: 617 calories

Total Fat: 24g

Cholesterol: 179mg

Sodium: 914mg

Total Carbohydrate: 58g

Protein: 42g

Fiber: 4g

171.   Chicken And Ham Lasagna

Serving: 12
Preparation Time: 25 Minutes
Cooking Time: 35 Minutes

Ingredients

3/4 pound fresh mushrooms, sliced

1 large onion, chopped

1 large green pepper, chopped

1/4 cup butter

1/2 cup all-purpose flour

1-2/3 cups whole milk

1 can (14-1/2 ounces) chicken broth

1 package (16 ounces) frozen chopped broccoli, thawed and drained

2/3 cup grated Parmesan cheese

1/2 teaspoon salt

1/4 to 1/2 teaspoon white pepper

1/8 teaspoon ground nutmeg

12 lasagna noodles, cooked and drained

2 cups cubed fully cooked ham

2 cups shredded Swiss cheese

2 cups cubed cooked chicken

Direction

In a large skillet, sauté the mushrooms, onion and green pepper in butter until tender. Stir in flour until blended. Gradually add milk and broth. Bring to a boil; cook and stir for 2 minutes or until thickened. Stir in the broccoli, Parmesan cheese, salt, pepper and nutmeg. Spread 2 cups broccoli mixture in a greased 13x9-in. baking dish. Top with four noodles, overlapping if needed. Layer with 2 cups broccoli mixture, 1-1/2 cups of ham, 2/3 cup Swiss cheese, four noodles, 2 cups broccoli mixture, chicken, 2/3 cup Swiss cheese, four noodles and remaining broccoli mixture, Swiss cheese and ham. Cover and bake at 350 degrees for 35-45 minutes or until heated through. Let stand for 15 minutes before cutting.

Nutrition:

Calories: 362 calories

Total Fat: 16g

Cholesterol: 68mg

Sodium: 754mg

Total Carbohydrate: 31g

Protein: 26g

Fiber: 3g

172. Chicken Broccoli Lasagna

Serving: 12
Preparation Time: 35 Minutes
Cooking Time: 40 Minutes

Ingredients

6 tablespoons butter, divided

1/4 cup all-purpose flour

2 cups whole milk

1 cup chicken broth

3 large eggs, lightly beaten

3/4 cup grated Parmesan cheese, divided

1 teaspoon salt, divided

Pinch ground nutmeg

Pinch cayenne pepper

1 cup chopped onion

1 garlic clove, minced

2 cups diced cooked chicken

1 package (16 ounces) frozen chopped broccoli, thawed and drained

1/2 cup shredded carrot

1/4 cup minced fresh parsley

1/4 teaspoon pepper

15 lasagna noodles, cooked and drained

4 cups shredded part-skim mozzarella cheese

Direction

In a large saucepan, melt 4 tablespoons butter; stir in flour until smooth.
Gradually add milk and broth; bring to a boil. Boil and stir for 2 minutes.
Whisk half into eggs; return all to pan. Cook and stir over low heat for about
1 minute or until mixture reaches at least 160 degrees. Remove from heat;
add 1/2 cup Parmesan, 1/2 teaspoon salt, nutmeg and cayenne. Set aside.
In a large skillet, sauté onion and garlic in remaining butter until tender. Add
the chicken, broccoli, carrot, parsley, pepper and remaining salt; cook for 3

minutes. Spread 1/2 cup of the Parmesan custard mixture into an ungreased 13x9-in. baking dish. Layer with a third of the noodles, half of the chicken mixture, 1/2 cup Parmesan custard, a third of the mozzarella cheese and 1 tablespoon Parmesan cheese. Repeat layers. Top with remaining noodles, mozzarella and Parmesan custard. Sprinkle with remaining Parmesan cheese. Bake, uncovered, at 350 degrees for 40-45 minutes or until bubbly. Let stand 10 minutes before serving.

Nutrition:

Calories: 408 calories

Total Fat: 20g

Cholesterol: 128mg

Sodium: 633mg

Total Carbohydrate: 32g

Protein: 25g

Fiber: 3g

173.   Chicken Cheese Lasagna

Serving: 12
Preparation Time: 25 Minutes
Cooking Time: 35 Minutes

Ingredients

1 medium onion, chopped

1/2 cup butter, cubed

1 garlic clove, minced

1/2 cup all-purpose flour

1 teaspoon salt

2 cups chicken broth

1-1/2 cups 2% milk

4 cups shredded part-skim mozzarella cheese, divided

1 cup grated Parmesan cheese, divided

1 teaspoon dried basil

1 teaspoon dried oregano

1/2 teaspoon white pepper

2 cups ricotta cheese

1 tablespoon minced fresh parsley

9 lasagna noodles, cooked and drained

2 packages (10 ounces each) frozen spinach, thawed and well drained

2 cups cubed cooked chicken

Direction

In a large saucepan, sauté onion in butter until tender. Add garlic; cook 1 minute longer. Stir in flour and salt until blended; cook until bubbly. Gradually stir in broth and milk. Bring to a boil; cook and stir for 1 minute or until thickened. Stir in 2 cups mozzarella, 1/2 cup Parmesan cheese, basil, oregano and pepper; set aside. In a large bowl, combine the ricotta cheese, parsley and remaining mozzarella; set aside. Spread one-quarter of the cheese sauce into a greased 13x9-in. baking dish; cover with one-third of the noodles. Layer with half of the ricotta mixture, half of the spinach and half of the chicken. Cover with one-quarter of the cheese sauce and one-third of the noodles. Repeat layers of ricotta mixture, spinach, chicken and one-quarter cheese sauce. Cover with remaining noodles and cheese sauce. Sprinkle with remaining Parmesan cheese. Bake at 350 degrees, uncovered, for 35-40 minutes. Let stand 15 minutes.

Nutrition:

Calories: 410 calories

Total Fat: 22g

Cholesterol: 87mg

Sodium: 830mg

Total Carbohydrate: 25g

Protein: 28g

Fiber: 2g

174.   Chicken Chili Lasagna

Serving: 12
Preparation Time: 35 Minutes
Cooking Time: 40 Minutes

Ingredients

6 ounces cream cheese, softened

1 medium onion, chopped

8 green onions, chopped

2 cups shredded Mexican cheese blend, divided

2 garlic cloves, minced

3/4 teaspoon ground cumin, divided

1/2 teaspoon minced fresh cilantro

3 cups cubed cooked chicken

1/4 cup butter

1/4 cup all-purpose flour

1-1/2 cups chicken broth

1 cup shredded Monterey Jack cheese

1 cup sour cream

1 can (4 ounces) chopped green chilies, drained

1/8 teaspoon dried thyme

1/8 teaspoon salt

1/8 teaspoon pepper

12 flour tortillas (6 inches), halved

Direction

In a large bowl, beat the cream cheese, onions, 1-1/2 cups Mexican-cheese blend, garlic, 1/4 teaspoon cumin and cilantro until blended. Stir in chicken; set aside. In a large saucepan, melt butter. Stir in flour until smooth; gradually add broth. Bring to a boil; cook and stir for 2 minutes or until thickened. Remove from the heat. Stir in Monterey Jack cheese, sour cream, chilies, thyme, salt, pepper and remaining cumin. Spread 1/2 cup of the cheese sauce in a greased 13x9-in. baking dish. Top with six tortilla halves, a third of the chicken mixture and a fourth of the cheese sauce. Repeat tortilla, chicken and cheese sauce layers twice. Top with remaining tortillas, cheese sauce and Mexican cheese. Cover and bake at 350 degrees for 30 minutes. Uncover; bake 10 minutes longer or until heated through. Let stand 5 minutes before cutting.

Nutrition:

Calories: 386 calories

Total Fat: 24g

Cholesterol: 88mg

Sodium: 688mg

Total Carbohydrate: 19g

Protein: 22g

Fiber: 1g

175. Chicken Curry Lasagna

Serving: 12
Preparation Time: 30 Minutes
Cooking Time: 40 Minutes

Ingredients

1 tablespoon canola oil

1 medium onion, chopped

4 teaspoons curry powder

3 garlic cloves, minced

1 can (6 ounces) tomato paste

2 cans (13.66 ounces each) coconut milk

1 pound (about 4 cups) shredded rotisserie chicken, skin removed

12 lasagna noodles, uncooked

2 cups part-skim ricotta cheese

2 large eggs

1/2 cup chopped fresh cilantro, divided

1 package (10 ounces) frozen chopped spinach, thawed and squeezed dry

1/2 teaspoon salt

1/4 teaspoon pepper

2 cups shredded part-skim mozzarella cheese

Lime wedges

Direction

Preheat oven to 350 degrees. In a large skillet, heat oil over medium-high heat. Add onion; cook and stir until softened, about 5 minutes. Add curry powder and garlic; cook 1 minute more. Stir in tomato paste; pour coconut milk into skillet. Bring to a boil. Reduce heat and simmer 5 minutes. Stir in cooked chicken. Meanwhile, cook lasagna noodles according to package directions. Drain. Combine ricotta, eggs, 1/4 cup cilantro, spinach and seasonings. Spread one-fourth of chicken mixture into a 13x9-in. baking dish coated with cooking spray. Layer with four noodles, half of ricotta mixture, one-fourth of chicken mixture and 1/2 cup mozzarella. Repeat layers. Top with remaining noodles, remaining chicken mixture and remaining mozzarella. Bake, uncovered, until bubbly, 40-45 minutes. Cool 10 minutes before cutting. Top with remaining cilantro; serve with lime wedges.

Nutrition:

Calories: 343 calories

Total Fat: 17g

Cholesterol: 68mg

Sodium: 322mg

Total Carbohydrate: 28g

Protein: 20g

Fiber: 2g

176. Chicken Lasagna Rolls

Serving: 5
Preparation Time: 45 Minutes
Cooking Time: 25 Minutes

Ingredients

1 medium onion, chopped

1/2 cup chopped sweet red pepper

1/2 cup chopped almonds

1/3 cup butter

1/2 cup cornstarch

1-1/2 teaspoons salt

2 cans (10-1/2 ounces each) condensed chicken broth, undiluted

2 cups chopped cooked chicken

1 package (10 ounces) frozen chopped spinach, thawed and well drained

1/4 teaspoon pepper

1/4 teaspoon ground nutmeg

10 lasagna noodles, cooked and drained

2 cups whole milk

1 cup shredded Swiss cheese, divided

1/4 cup dry white wine or water

Direction

Preheat oven to 350 degrees. In a large saucepan, sauté onion, red pepper and almonds in butter until onion is tender and almonds are toasted. Stir in cornstarch and salt until blended. Stir in broth. Bring to a boil; cook and stir 2 minutes or until thickened. Transfer half of the sauce to a large bowl; stir in chicken, spinach, pepper and nutmeg. Spread about 3 tablespoons over each lasagna noodle. Roll up and place seam side down in a greased 11x7-in. baking dish. Add milk, 1/2 cup Swiss cheese and wine to remaining sauce. Cook and stir over medium heat until thickened and bubbly. Pour over roll-ups. Bake, uncovered, 20-25 minutes. Sprinkle with remaining cheese; bake 5 minutes longer or until cheese is melted.

Nutrition:

Calories: 717 calories

Total Fat: 34g

Cholesterol: 116mg

Sodium: 1404mg

Total Carbohydrate: 63g

Protein: 40g

Fiber: 6g

177.   Contadina Butternut Squash Lasagna

Serving: 8
Preparation Time: 10 Minutes
Cooking Time: 1 h 10 Minutes

Ingredients

12 dry lasagna noodles

3 tablespoons olive oil

1 cup chopped onion

1 tablespoon minced garlic

1 pound butternut squash, cut into 1-inch cubes

1 (28 ounce) can CONTADINA® Crushed Tomatoes

1 (15 ounce) can CONTADINA® Tomato Sauce

1/4 cup chopped fresh basil

1 tablespoon chopped fresh rosemary

1 teaspoon balsamic vinegar

1 teaspoon sugar

2 cups ricotta cheese

1 egg

4 tablespoons grated Parmesan cheese, divided

3 cups shredded mozzarella cheese

Direction

Preheat oven to 375 degrees F. Spray a 13x9-inch baking dish with non-stick cooking spray; set aside. Cook lasagna noodles according to package directions; drain.

Heat oil in large saucepan over medium heat; cook onion and garlic 3 minutes, stirring frequently.

Add squash, crushed tomatoes, tomato sauce, basil, rosemary, balsamic vinegar and sugar. Bring to a boil; reduce heat. Simmer 12 minutes or until squash is tender.

Remove from heat. Lightly mash squash with a potato masher.

Stir together ricotta, egg and 2 Tbsp. Parmesan cheese in a medium bowl; set aside.

Layer 4 lasagna noodles, 1/3 sauce, 1/3 ricotta mixture and 1/3 mozzarella cheese.

Repeat 2 more times ending with ricotta and mozzarella.

Cover with foil. Bake 45 minutes. Remove foil. Sprinkle with remaining 2 Tbsp. Parmesan cheese. Bake, uncovered, 10 minutes or until cheese is lightly browned.

Remove from oven. Let rest 5 to 10 minutes. Sprinkle with additional chopped basil before serving, if desired.

Nutrition:

Calories: 470 calories

Total Fat: 18.9 g

Cholesterol: 72 mg

Sodium: 880 mg

Total Carbohydrate: 49.4 g

Protein: 27.2 g

178. Crab Lasagna Rollups

Serving: 6
Preparation Time: 20 Minutes
Cooking Time: 30 Minutes

Ingredients

2 cups (16 ounces) 1% cottage cheese

1/2 cup egg substitute

1/4 cup grated Parmesan cheese

2 tablespoons Italian seasoning

2 tablespoons minced fresh parsley

1 teaspoon dried oregano

1/2 teaspoon dried basil

1/2 teaspoon dried thyme

1/4 teaspoon garlic powder

1 package (8 ounces) imitation crabmeat, flaked

12 lasagna noodles, cooked and drained

2 cans (8 ounces each) no-salt-added tomato sauce

Direction

In a bowl, combine the first nine ingredients. Add crab; mix well. Place about 1/3 cup on each noodle; roll up. Place seam side down in a 13-in. x 9-in. baking dish coated with cooking spray. Top with tomato sauce. Cover and bake at 350 degrees for 30-40 minutes or until heated through.

Nutrition:

Calories: 198 calories

Total Fat: 3g

Cholesterol: 13mg

Sodium: 755mg

Total Carbohydrate: 23g

Protein: 19g

Fiber: 1g

179.   Creamy Broccoli Lasagna

Serving: 12
Preparation Time: 15 Minutes
Cooking Time: 35 Minutes

Ingredients
9 uncooked lasagna noodles
1/4 cup chopped onion
1/4 cup butter
1/4 cup all-purpose flour
2 teaspoons chicken bouillon granules
3/4 teaspoon garlic salt
1/4 teaspoon pepper
1/4 teaspoon dried thyme
2-1/2 cups milk
6 cups broccoli florets
1-1/2 cups (12 ounces) 4% cottage cheese
2 jars (4-1/2 ounces each) sliced mushrooms, drained
2 packages (6 ounces each) slices Swiss cheese
Direction
Preheat oven to 350 degrees. Cook noodles according to package directions.
Meanwhile, in a large saucepan, sauté onion in butter until tender. Add flour,
bouillon, garlic salt, pepper and thyme; stir until smooth. Gradually add
milk. Bring to a boil; cook and stir 2 minutes or until thickened. Add
broccoli; cook 3-5 minutes. Stir in cottage cheese and mushrooms. Drain
noodles. In a greased 13x9-in. baking dish, layer three noodles, a third of
the sauce and a third of the Swiss cheese. Repeat layers twice. Bake,
uncovered, 35-40 minutes or until bubbly and broccoli is tender. Let stand
10 minutes before cutting.
Nutrition:
Calories: 291 calories
Total Fat: 15g
Cholesterol: 49mg
Sodium: 542mg
Total Carbohydrate: 23g
Protein: 17g
Fiber: 2g

180. Creamy Lasagna Casserole

Serving: 2 casseroles (4-6each).
Preparation Time: 30 Minutes
Cooking Time: 25 Minutes

Ingredients
2 pounds ground beef
1 can (29 ounces) tomato sauce
1 teaspoon salt
1/2 teaspoon pepper
1/2 teaspoon garlic powder
6 ounces cream cheese, softened
2 cups (16 ounces) sour cream
2 cups shredded cheddar cheese, divided
4 green onions, chopped
12 to 14 lasagna noodles, cooked and drained
Direction
In a Dutch oven, cook beef over medium heat until no longer pink; drain.
Add the tomato sauce, salt, pepper and garlic powder. Bring to a boil.
Reduce heat; simmer, uncovered, for 15 minutes. In a large bowl, beat
cream cheese until smooth. Add the sour cream, 1 cup cheddar cheese and
onions; mix well. Spread about 1/2 cup meat sauce into each of two greased
8-in. square baking dishes. Place two to three noodles in each dish,
trimming to fit as necessary. Top each with about 1/2 cup cream cheese
mixture and 2/3 cup meat sauce. Repeat layers twice. Sprinkle 1/2 cup
cheddar cheese over each. Cover and freeze one casserole for up to 1
month. Bake remaining casserole, uncovered, at 350 degrees for 25-30
minutes or until bubbly and heated through. Let stand for 15 minutes before
cutting. To use frozen casserole: Thaw in the refrigerator for 18 hours.
Remove from the refrigerator 30 minutes before baking. Bake, uncovered, at
350 degrees for 40-50 minutes or until heated through.
Nutrition:
Calories:
Total Fat: g
Cholesterol: mg
Sodium: mg
Total Carbohydrate: g
Protein: g
Fiber: g

181. Donna Lasagna

Serving: 12
Preparation Time: 40 Minutes
Cooking Time: 60 Minutes

Ingredients

1 pound lean ground beef (90% lean)

8 ounces Johnsonville TM ; Ground Mild or Hot Italian sausage

1 can (15 ounces) tomato puree

2 cans (6 ounces each) tomato paste

3 tablespoons dried parsley flakes, divided

2 tablespoons sugar

1 tablespoon dried basil

1-1/2 teaspoons salt, divided

1 garlic clove, minced

2 large eggs, lightly beaten

3 cups (24 ounces) cream-style cottage cheese

1/2 cup grated Parmesan cheese

1/2 teaspoon pepper

9 lasagna noodles, cooked and drained

4 cups shredded part-skim mozzarella cheese

Direction

In a Dutch oven, cook beef and sausage over medium heat until no longer
pink; drain. Add the tomato puree, tomato paste, 1 tablespoon parsley,
sugar, basil, 1 teaspoon salt and garlic. Bring to a boil. Reduce heat;
simmer, uncovered, for 30 minutes. In a large bowl, combine the eggs,
cottage cheese, Parmesan cheese, pepper, and remaining parsley and salt.
Spread 1/2 cup meat mixture in a greased 13x9-in. baking dish. Layer with
three noodles, a third of the cheese mixture, 1-1/3 cups mozzarella cheese
and a third of remaining meat sauce. Repeat layers twice. Bake at 350
degrees for 1 hour or until a thermometer reads 160 degrees. Let stand for
15 minutes before cutting.

Nutrition:

Calories: 377 calories

Total Fat: 18g

Cholesterol: 102mg

Sodium: 925mg

Total Carbohydrate: 24g

Protein: 29g

Fiber: 2g

182.   Easy Dutch Oven Cheese Lasagna

Serving: 12
Preparation Time: 15 Minutes
Cooking Time: 1 h 15 Minutes

Ingredients

1 (32 ounce) jar spaghetti sauce

15 lasagna noodles

2 cups broccoli florets

2 cups cauliflower florets

1 cup green peas

1 cup corn

2 cups shredded mozzarella cheese

1 cup shredded Cheddar cheese

Direction

Pour about 1/2 cup of spaghetti sauce into the bottom of a large, cast-iron Dutch oven with lid. Spread the sauce around evenly.

Place down a layer of three lasagna noodles, and spread about 3/4 cup of spaghetti sauce over them. Lay in the broccoli and sprinkle with 2/3 cup of mozzarella cheese. Repeat this layering of noodles, sauce, vegetables, and cheese using the cauliflower, green peas, and corn.

Cover the corn with the last three remaining lasagna noodles, and spread the remaining spaghetti sauce on top. Sprinkle with the Cheddar cheese.

Place the lid on the Dutch oven, and place 12 hot coals underneath and 12 coals on top. Cook for 75 minutes or until noodles are soft and tender. Remove the coals, and allow to stand for about 10 minutes to firm up a bit before serving.

Nutrition:

Calories: 288 calories

Total Fat: 9.1 g

Cholesterol: 23 mg

Sodium: 495 mg

Total Carbohydrate: 38.8 g

Protein: 14.1 g

183. Easy Lasagna

Serving: 12
Preparation Time: 5 Minutes
Cooking Time: 45 Minutes

Ingredients

1-1/2 cups 4% cottage cheese

1 large egg

1/4 cup grated Parmesan cheese

1 tablespoon minced fresh parsley or 1 teaspoon dried parsley flakes

1/2 teaspoon dried oregano

1/4 teaspoon dried basil

9 lasagna noodles, cooked, rinsed and drained

4 cups Three-Meat Sauce

2 cups shredded part-skim mozzarella cheese

Direction

In a large bowl, combine the cottage cheese, egg, Parmesan cheese, parsley, oregano and basil. In a greased 13x9-in. baking dish, layer a third of the noodles, sauce, cottage cheese mixture and mozzarella. Repeat layers twice. Cover and bake at 350 degrees for 30 minutes; uncover and bake 15-20 minutes longer or until bubbly. Let stand for 15 minutes before cutting.

Nutrition:

Calories: 282 calories

Total Fat: 13g

Cholesterol: 67mg

Sodium: 665mg

Total Carbohydrate: 20g

Protein: 20g

Fiber: 1g

184. Easy Lasagna I

Serving: 8
Preparation Time: 35 Minutes
Cooking Time: 1 hours

Ingredients

1 pound lean ground beef

1 onion, chopped

1 (4.5 ounce) can mushrooms, drained

1 (28 ounce) jar spaghetti sauce

1 (16 ounce) package cottage cheese

1 pint part-skim ricotta cheese

1/4 cup grated Parmesan cheese

2 eggs

1 (16 ounce) package lasagna noodles

8 ounces shredded mozzarella cheese

Direction

Preheat oven to 350 degrees F (175 degrees C).

In a large skillet, cook and stir ground beef until brown. Add mushrooms and onions; sauté until onions are transparent. Stir in pasta sauce, and heat through.

In a medium size bowl, combine cottage cheese, ricotta cheese, grated Parmesan cheese, and eggs.

Spread a thin layer of the meat sauce in the bottom of a 13x9 inch pan. Layer with uncooked lasagna noodles, cheese mixture, mozzarella cheese, and meat sauce. Continue layering until all ingredients are used, reserving 1/2 cup mozzarella. Cover pan with aluminum foil.

Bake in preheated oven for 45 minutes. Uncover, and top with remaining half cup of mozzarella cheese. Bake for an additional 15 minutes. Remove from oven, and let stand 10 to 15 minutes before serving.

Nutrition:

Calories: 702 calories

Total Fat: 30.3 g

Cholesterol: 142 mg

Sodium: 1058 mg

Total Carbohydrate: 62.5 g

Protein: 44.2 g

185. Easy Mexican Lasagna

Serving: 12
Preparation Time: 15 Minutes
Cooking Time: 01 h 35 Minutes

Ingredients

1 pound lean ground beef (90% lean)

1 can (16 ounces) refried beans

2 teaspoons dried oregano

1 teaspoon ground cumin

3/4 teaspoon garlic powder

12 uncooked lasagna noodles

2-1/2 cups water

2-1/2 cups picante sauce or salsa

2 cups sour cream

3/4 cup finely sliced green onions

1 can (2-1/4 ounces) sliced ripe olives, drained

1 cup shredded Monterey Jack cheese

Direction

Combine beef, beans, oregano, cumin and garlic powder. Place four of the uncooked lasagna noodles in a 13x9-in. baking dish. Spread half the beef mixture over the noodles. Top with four more noodles and the remaining beef mixture. Cover and remaining noodles. Combine water and picante sauce. Pour over all. Cover tightly with foil; bake at 350 degrees for 1-1/2 hours or until noodles are tender. Combine sour cream, onions and olives. Spoon over casserole; top with cheese. Bake, uncovered, until cheese is melted, about 5 minutes.

Nutrition:

Calories: 325 calories

Total Fat: 14g

Cholesterol: 57mg

Sodium: 473mg

Total Carbohydrate: 30g

Protein: 17g

Fiber: 3g

186.   Easy Passover Lasagna

Serving: 10
Preparation Time: 15 Minutes
Cooking Time: 45 Minutes

Ingredients

28 ounces ricotta cheese

3 eggs

8 matzah sheets, or more as needed

3 (32 ounce) jars marinara sauce (such as Classico® Tomato and Basil)

2 (16 ounce) packages shredded mozzarella cheese

Direction

Preheat oven to 350 degrees F (175 degrees C).

Beat ricotta cheese and eggs together in a bowl.

Briefly pass each matzah sheet under warm running water; layer moistened sheets on a plate.

Spread a thin layer of marinara sauce in the bottom of a deep 11x15-inch baking dish; top with a layer of moistened matzah sheets, breaking pieces as needed to completely cover marinara. Spread a layer of ricotta mixture over matzah mixture. Sprinkle mozzarella cheese over ricotta mixture layer. Repeat layering with remaining ingredients, ending with a layer of matzah, marinara, and mozzarella cheese, respectively.

Bake in the preheated oven until cheese is bubbling and browned, about 45 minutes.

Nutrition:

Calories: 683 calories

Total Fat: 29.5 g

Cholesterol: 144 mg

Sodium: 1784 mg

Total Carbohydrate: 62.9 g

Protein: 40.1 g

187.   Easy Seafood Lasagna

Serving: 12
Preparation Time: 15 Minutes
Cooking Time: 50 Minutes

Ingredients

3/4 cup chopped onion

2 tablespoons butter

1 package (8 ounces) cream cheese, cubed

1-1/2 cups (12 ounces) 4% cottage cheese

1 egg, lightly beaten

2 teaspoons dried basil

1 teaspoon salt

1/4 teaspoon pepper

1 can (10-3/4 ounces) condensed cream of shrimp soup, undiluted

1 can (10-3/4 ounces) condensed cream of mushroom soup, undiluted

1/2 cup white wine or chicken broth

1/2 cup milk

2 packages (8 ounces each) imitation crabmeat, flaked

1 can (6 ounces) small shrimp, rinsed and drained

9 lasagna noodles, cooked and drained

1/2 cup grated Parmesan cheese

3/4 cup shredded Monterey Jack cheese

Direction

In a large skillet, sauté onion in butter until tender. Reduce heat. Add cream cheese; cook and stir until melted and smooth. Stir in the cottage cheese, egg, basil, salt and pepper. Remove from the heat and set aside. In a large bowl, combine the soups, wine or broth, milk, crab and shrimp. Arrange three noodles in a greased 13-in. x 9-in. baking dish. Spread with a third of cottage cheese mixture and a third of the seafood mixture. Repeat layers twice. Sprinkle with Parmesan cheese. Cover and bake at 350 degrees for 40 minutes. Uncover; sprinkle with the Monterey Jack cheese. Bake 10 minutes longer or until cheese is melted and lasagna is bubbly. Let stand for 15 minutes before serving.

Nutrition:

Calories: 314 calories

Total Fat: 16g

Cholesterol: 96mg

Sodium: 1132mg

Total Carbohydrate: 24g

Protein: 17g

Fiber: 1g

188.   Easy Vegetarian Red Beans Lasagna

Serving: 4
Preparation Time: 20 Minutes
Cooking Time: 35 Minutes

Ingredients

1 tablespoon olive oil

1 small onion, chopped

1 clove garlic, minced

1 (15 ounce) can red beans, drained

1 (14.5 ounce) can diced tomatoes, drained

1/2 red bell pepper, chopped

1 teaspoon dried basil

1 teaspoon dried oregano

salt and pepper to taste

3 tablespoons butter

3 tablespoons all-purpose flour

1 1/2 cups cold milk

1/2 cup grated Parmesan cheese

4 no-boil lasagna noodles

4 ounces shredded Gruyere cheese

Direction

Preheat oven to 350 degrees F (175 degrees C).

Heat the olive oil in a skillet over medium heat, and cook the onion until tender. Mix in garlic, and cook until heated through. Mix in red beans, tomatoes, and red bell pepper. Season with basil, oregano, salt, and pepper. Continue cooking 10 minutes, stirring occasionally.

Melt the butter in a saucepan over medium heat, and gradually mix in flour until smooth. Slowly stir in the milk. Mix in Parmesan cheese, and continue to cook and stir until slightly thickened.

Spread 1/2 the red bean mixture in a 9x9 inch casserole dish, and top with 2 lasagna noodles. Layer with remaining bean mixture and remaining noodles. Cover with the sauce, and top with Gruyere cheese.

Bake 20 minutes in the preheated oven, or until lightly browned.

Nutrition:

Calories: 496 calories

Total Fat: 27 g

Cholesterol: 71 mg

Sodium: 800 mg

Total Carbohydrate: 39.9 g

Protein: 23.9 g

189. Enchilada Lasagna

Serving: 10
Preparation Time: 15 Minutes
Cooking Time: 30 Minutes

Ingredients

2 pounds ground beef

1 medium onion, chopped

2 garlic cloves, minced

1 can (10-3/4 ounces) condensed tomato soup, undiluted

1 cup picante sauce or salsa

1 can (16 ounces) refried beans

10 flour tortillas (6 inches)

4 cups shredded cheddar cheese

Direction

In a skillet, cook ground beef, onion and garlic until the meat is browned and onion is tender; drain. Stir in tomato soup, picante sauce or salsa and refried beans. Heat thoroughly. Arrange five tortillas in a 12x8x2-in. baking dish, tearing tortillas as needed to cover the bottom. Layer with half of the meat mixture and half of the cheese. Repeat layers using remaining tortillas, meat mixture and cheese. Bake at 350 degrees for 30 minutes or until heated through. Let stand a few minutes before serving.

Nutrition:

Calories: 469 calories

Total Fat: 25g

Cholesterol: 96mg

Sodium: 976mg

Total Carbohydrate: 29g

Protein: 32g

Fiber: 3g

190.   Fabulous Foolproof Lasagna

Serving: 8
Preparation Time: 15 Minutes
Cooking Time: 45 Minutes

Ingredients

1 pound Italian sausage, casings removed

1 pint ricotta cheese

1 egg, lightly beaten

1/2 teaspoon dried basil

1/2 teaspoon dried thyme

1/2 teaspoon garlic powder

1/2 teaspoon dried oregano

8 ounces shredded mozzarella cheese, divided

1 (16 ounce) jar spaghetti sauce

12 no-boil lasagna noodles

3/4 cup grated Parmesan cheese

Direction

Preheat oven to 350 degrees F (175 degrees C).

In a medium skillet over medium heat, cook the sausage until brown and the juices run clear. Drain and set aside.

In a small bowl, combine ricotta, egg, basil, thyme, garlic powder, oregano and half the shredded mozzarella. Mix well, and set aside.

Coat the bottom of a 9x13 baking dish with a little of the spaghetti sauce. Place three noodles in the bottom of the pan, not touching. Spread a layer of the ricotta mixture, a layer of sausage, and a layer of spaghetti sauce over the noodles. Repeat three more times. Top with the reserved mozzarella and Parmesan. Cover with foil.

Bake in preheated oven 30 minutes, remove foil and bake 15 minutes more, until golden and bubbly.

Nutrition:

Calories: 462 calories

Total Fat: 25.9 g

Cholesterol: 95 mg

Sodium: 1094 mg

Total Carbohydrate: 26.9 g

Protein: 29.6 g

191.   Favorite Skillet Lasagna

Serving: 5
Preparation Time: 10 Minutes
Cooking Time: 20 Minutes

Ingredients

1/2 pound Italian turkey sausage links, casings removed

1 small onion, chopped

1 jar (14 ounces) spaghetti sauce

2 cups uncooked whole wheat egg noodles

1 cup water

1/2 cup chopped zucchini

1/2 cup fat-free ricotta cheese

2 tablespoons grated Parmesan cheese

1 tablespoon minced fresh parsley or 1 teaspoon dried parsley flakes

1/2 cup shredded part-skim mozzarella cheese

Direction

In a large nonstick skillet, cook sausage and onion over medium heat until no longer pink, breaking up sausage into crumbles; drain. Stir in spaghetti sauce, noodles, water and zucchini. Bring to a boil. Reduce heat; simmer, covered, 8-10 minutes or until noodles are tender, stirring occasionally. In a small bowl, combine ricotta cheese, Parmesan cheese and parsley. Drop by tablespoonfuls over pasta mixture. Sprinkle with mozzarella cheese; cook, covered, 3-5 minutes longer or until cheese is melted.

Nutrition:

Calories: 250 calories

Total Fat: 10g

Cholesterol: 41mg

Sodium: 783mg

Total Carbohydrate: 24g

Protein: 17g

Fiber: 3g

192.   Fiesta Surprise

Serving: 8-10
Preparation Time: 25 Minutes
Cooking Time: 45 Minutes

Ingredients

1-1/2 pounds ground beef

1 medium onion, chopped

1 envelope taco seasoning

1 cup water

1/2 cup taco sauce

10 corn tortillas (6 inches)

2 packages (10 ounces each) frozen chopped spinach, thawed and partially drained

3 cups shredded Monterey Jack cheese

1/2 cup chopped fully cooked ham

1 cup sour cream

Direction

In a skillet, cook beef and onion over medium heat until meat is no longer pink; drain. Stir in taco seasoning and water. Cover and simmer for 10 minutes. Pour 1/4 cup taco sauce in a 13x9-in. baking dish; coat five tortillas on both sides with the sauce. Overlap the tortillas to make bottom layer. Stir one package of spinach into the beef mixture; spoon over the tortillas. Top with half of the cheese. Cover with remaining tortillas, overlapping as needed. Spread with remaining taco sauce. Sprinkle with ham; cover with sour cream. Sprinkle remaining spinach over top; cover with remaining cheese. Bake at 350 degrees for 45 minutes or until heated through. Let stand for 5-10 minutes before serving.

Nutrition:

Calories:

Total Fat: g

Cholesterol: mg

Sodium: mg

Total Carbohydrate: g

Protein: g

Fiber: g

193. Vegetarian Baked Pasta

Serving: 8
Preparation Time: 20 Minutes
Cooking Time: 45 Minutes

Ingredients

1 pound penne pasta

2 tablespoons olive oil

8 ounces portobello mushrooms, cut into 1/2 inch pieces

1 teaspoon dried basil

1 teaspoon dried oregano

2 cloves garlic, minced

1 (28 ounce) jar spaghetti sauce

4 cups shredded mozzarella cheese

8 ounces Gorgonzola cheese, crumbled

Direction

Bring a large pot of lightly salted water to a boil. Add pasta and cook for 8 to 10 minutes or until al dente; drain. Pour a glass of ice water over the pasta to stop the cooking, but do not rinse thoroughly.

Preheat oven to 350 degrees F (175 degrees C). Coat a 9 x 13 glass pan with olive oil. Heat 2 tablespoons olive oil in large skillet. Add mushrooms. Cook for 2 minutes then add basil, oregano and garlic and cook 1 minute more. Add sauce to mushroom mixture and stir.

To assemble, pour enough sauce in the bottom of the pan to cover. Combine the remaining sauce and the pasta. Place one-third of sauced noodles on top of sauce in pan. Top with 1 cup of mozzarella and one-half of the gorgonzola. Repeat for a second layer. Put the final third of the noodles in the pan and top with the final 2 cups of mozzarella.

Bake for 30 to 45 minutes, or until cheese is browned. Serve.

Nutrition:

Calories: 571 calories

Total Fat: 24.4 g

Cholesterol: 68 mg

Sodium: 1036 mg

Total Carbohydrate: 58.3 g

Protein: 29.8 g

194.   Vegetarian Four Cheese Lasagna

Serving: 8
Preparation Time: 15 Minutes
Cooking Time: 1 hours

Ingredients

2 cups peeled and diced pumpkin

1 eggplant, sliced into 1/2 inch rounds

5 tomatoes

1 pint ricotta cheese

9 ounces crumbled feta cheese

2/3 cup pesto

2 eggs, beaten

salt and pepper to taste

1 (15 ounce) can tomato sauce

fresh pasta sheets

1 1/3 cups shredded mozzarella cheese

1 cup grated Parmesan cheese

Direction

Preheat oven to 350 degrees F (175 degrees C).

Place pumpkin on a baking sheet and roast in oven until browned and tender, about 30 minutes. Meanwhile, grill eggplant on a charcoal grill or fry in a skillet, turning once, until charred and tender, 10 to 15 minutes. Halve tomatoes and place on baking sheet in oven for last 15 minutes of pumpkin time; cook until tender and wrinkly.

In a medium bowl, stir together ricotta, feta, pesto, eggs, salt and pepper until well mixed. Fold roasted pumpkin into ricotta mixture.

Spoon half of the tomato sauce into a 9x13 baking dish. Lay two pasta sheets over the sauce. Arrange a single layer of eggplant slices over pasta and top with half the ricotta mixture. Cover with two more pasta sheets. Arrange the roasted tomatoes evenly over the sheets and spoon the remaining half the ricotta mixture over the tomatoes. Sprinkle with half the mozzarella. Top with remaining two sheets of pasta. Pour remaining tomato sauce over all and sprinkle with remaining mozzarella and Parmesan.

Bake in preheated oven 30 to 40 minutes, until golden and bubbly.

Nutrition:

Calories: 451 calories

Total Fat: 29.5 g

Cholesterol: 124 mg

Sodium: 1176 mg

Total Carbohydrate: 20.4 g

Protein: 28.8 g

195.   Vegetarian Lentil Spaghetti

Serving: 4
Preparation Time: 10 Minutes
Cooking Time: 40 Minutes

Ingredients
1/4 cup dried brown lentils, rinsed and drained
1 (15 ounce) can stewed tomatoes, undrained
1 (15 ounce) can artichoke hearts in water
1/4 teaspoon cayenne pepper, divided
1/4 cup water
3 tablespoons olive oil, divided
1/4 pound thin spaghetti
4 green onions, chopped
1/2 teaspoon sesame seeds
salt and pepper to taste
Direction
Place the lentils, tomatoes and artichokes (with the liquid from the cans),
1/8 teaspoon cayenne pepper and the water into a large saucepan. Bring to
a boil. Reduce heat to low and simmer until lentils are tender, about 20
minutes.
Meanwhile, bring a large pot of lightly salted water and 1 tablespoon of the
olive oil to a boil. Add spaghetti and cook for 8 to 10 minutes or until al
dente; drain. Return pasta to pot and cover to keep warm.
Heat remaining 2 tablespoons olive oil in a small skillet over medium heat
and cook green onions for about 3 minutes. Add 1/8 teaspoon cayenne
pepper and sesame seeds and cook until the seeds are lightly browned,
about 2 minutes. Set aside.
Add the lentil mixture to the pot of pasta and toss to distribute evenly. Add
the green onion mixture and toss lightly again. Season with salt and pepper
to taste.
Nutrition:
Calories: 329 calories
Total Fat: 11.1 g
Cholesterol: 0 mg
Sodium: 883 mg
Total Carbohydrate: 47.5 g
Protein: 11.9 g

196. **Vegetarian Lime Orzo**

Serving: 4
Preparation Time: 35 Minutes
Cooking Time: 17 Minutes

Ingredients
2 tablespoons olive oil
2 cloves garlic, minced
2 cups orzo pasta
1 zucchini, peeled and shredded
1 carrot, peeled and shredded
1 (16 ounce) can stewed tomatoes, undrained
1 (14 ounce) can vegetable broth
1 teaspoon Italian seasoning
1 teaspoon dried basil leaves
salt and black pepper to taste
1/4 cup chopped green onions
1/4 cup chopped fresh parsley
2 teaspoons grated lime zest
2 tablespoons lime juice
1/2 cup grated Parmesan cheese for topping
Direction
Heat the olive oil in a large skillet over medium-high heat. Stir in the garlic
and orzo pasta; cook and stir until pasta turns a light, golden color, about 5
minutes. Stir in zucchini and carrots; cook until vegetables soften, about 2
minutes. Stir in the tomatoes, vegetable broth, Italian seasoning, and basil.
Season with salt and pepper to taste. Reduce heat to medium. Cover, and
simmer until almost all liquid is absorbed, about 10 minutes. Stir in the
green onions, parsley, lime zest, and lime juice. Remove from heat, cool
slightly, and serve sprinkled with Parmesan cheese.
Nutrition:
Calories: 535 calories
Total Fat: 12.3 g
Cholesterol: 11 mg
Sodium: 579 mg
Total Carbohydrate: 87.4 g
Protein: 20.9 g

197. Vegetarian Phad Thai

Serving: 8
Preparation Time: 20 Minutes
Cooking Time: 20 Minutes

Ingredients

1 pound dried rice noodles

2 tablespoons vegetable oil

4 eggs, beaten

2 tablespoons peanut oil

1 1/2 cups peanut butter

1/3 cup water

1/3 cup soy sauce

1 cup milk

1 1/4 cups brown sugar

1/3 cup lemon juice

2 tablespoons garlic powder

1 tablespoon paprika

cayenne pepper to taste

1 pound mung bean sprouts

1 cup shredded carrots

1/4 cup chopped green onions

1/2 cup chopped, unsalted dry-roasted peanuts

1 lime, cut into wedges

Direction

Submerge the rice noodles in a large bowl of hot water for about an hour.

Pour 1/2 tablespoon of oil into a large skillet, and add eggs. Scramble into medium-sized pieces, and transfer to plate. Set aside.

In a saucepan, mix together peanut oil, peanut butter, water, soy sauce, milk, brown sugar, and lemon juice. Season with garlic powder and paprika. Heat until sauce is smooth. Season liberally with cayenne pepper.

Drain noodles; noodles should be very flexible, but still relatively firm. Heat remaining 1 1/2 tablespoons vegetable oil in a large saucepan or wok. Cook noodles in oil, stirring constantly, until they are tender, about 2 minutes. Stir in peanut sauce, sprouts, carrots, scallions, ground peanuts, and the scrambled eggs. Continue to cook over low heat until vegetables are crisp-tender, about 5 minutes. Serve immediately, garnished with lime wedges.

Nutrition:

Calories: 830 calories

Total Fat: 39.4 g

Cholesterol: 95 mg

Sodium: 999 mg

Total Carbohydrate: 103.6 g

Protein: 23.6 g

198. Vegetarian Slow Cooker Meal

Serving: 6
Preparation Time: 5 Minutes
Cooking Time: 5 hours

Ingredients

1 (32 fluid ounce) container vegetable broth

1 (16 ounce) package frozen cheese-filled tortellini

1 (8 ounce) package cream cheese, cut into pieces

1 (8 ounce) package fresh spinach

1 cup sliced crimini ('baby bella') mushrooms

Direction

Stir vegetable broth, tortellini, cream cheese, spinach, and mushrooms
together in a slow cooker.

Cook on Low for 5 to 6 hours.

Nutrition:

Calories: 398 calories

Total Fat: 20 g

Cholesterol: 74 mg

Sodium: 733 mg

Total Carbohydrate: 40.8 g

Protein: 15.5 g

199.   Vegetarian White Bean Alfredo With Linguine

Serving: 6
Preparation Time: 15 Minutes
Cooking Time: 15 Minutes

Ingredients

1 (16 ounce) package linguine pasta

1/4 cup butter

3 cloves garlic, minced

2 cups cooked navy beans, rinsed and drained

1 1/2 cups soy milk

1 cup asparagus, cut into 1/2-inch pieces

salt and black pepper to taste

Direction

Fill a large pot with lightly salted water, and bring to a boil over high heat. Cook pasta in boiling water, stirring occasionally, until the pasta has cooked through, about 11 minutes. Drain well.

Meanwhile, melt the butter in a large saucepan over medium heat. Stir in the garlic, and cook until golden brown, about 5 minutes. Add 2/3 cup of the beans and 1/2 cup of soy milk; mash with the back of a spoon or a potato masher to create a thick paste. Stir in the remaining soy milk to create a thick sauce. Mix in the remaining beans and asparagus; simmer until asparagus is tender. Season to taste with salt and pepper. Toss pasta with the sauce, and serve.

Nutrition:

Calories: 474 calories

Total Fat: 10.9 g

Cholesterol: 20 mg

Sodium: 481 mg

Total Carbohydrate: 77.4 g

Protein: 19.2 g

200.   Vegetarian Whole Wheat Pasta With Broccoli And Gorgonzola

Serving: 1
Preparation Time: 5 Minutes
Cooking Time: 23 Minutes

Ingredients

2 ounces whole-wheat spaghetti

3 tablespoons crumbled Gorgonzola cheese

2 tablespoons sour cream

1 teaspoon butter

1 small onion, chopped

1 1/2 cups broccoli florets

1/2 cup water

1/2 teaspoon vegetable stock powder

salt and freshly ground black pepper to taste

1 pinch ground nutmeg

1 teaspoon lemon juice, or to taste

1 teaspoon chopped almonds

Direction

Bring a large pot of lightly salted water to a boil. Cook spaghetti in the boiling water, stirring occasionally, until tender yet firm to the bite according to package instructions, about 12 minutes. Drain.

Mix gorgonzola and sour cream together in a small bowl.

Heat butter in a skillet over medium heat while spaghetti is cooking. Add onion; cook until soft and translucent, about 5 minutes. Add broccoli, water, vegetable stock powder, salt, pepper, and nutmeg and cook until broccoli is soft, about 15 minutes. Puree broccoli mixture with an immersion blender until smooth.

Stir in gorgonzola-cream mixture and heat until sauce almost boils, 3 to 5 minutes. Season with lemon juice and pour over spaghetti. Sprinkle with almonds.

Nutrition:

Calories: 502 calories

Total Fat: 21.9 g

Cholesterol: 57 mg

Sodium: 576 mg

Total Carbohydrate: 60.9 g

Protein: 21.2 g

201.   Veggie Lasagna

Serving: 6
Preparation Time: 25 Minutes
Cooking Time: 45 Minutes

Ingredients

1 medium onion, finely diced

2 cloves garlic, minced

1 teaspoon Spectrum® Canola Oil

1 (8 ounce) container ricotta cheese

1/2 teaspoon salt

1 teaspoon ground black pepper

1 teaspoon oregano

1 tablespoon all-purpose flour

1/2 cup Europe's Best® Chefs Spinach, chopped and squeezed

1 (340 gram) package Yves Veggie Cuisine® Original Veggie Ground Round

5 cups tomato basil pasta sauce, divided

9 oven-ready lasagna noodles

3 cups shredded mozzarella cheese

Direction

Preheat oven to 350 degrees F (175 degrees C). Coat a 9 x13-inch (33 x 23 cm) lasagna pan lightly with oil.

Sauté onions and garlic in oil over medium heat. Set aside to cool.

In a bowl mix ricotta cheese or tofu with salt, pepper, oregano, flour, spinach and sautéed onions.

In another bowl mix Veggie Ground Round with 3 cups tomato sauce.

Layering: Spread 1/2 cup of the reserved tomato sauce on the bottom of pan and set 3 lasagna noodles in the sauce. Cover noodles with half of the Veggie Ground Round mixture and 1 cup of shredded cheese. Arrange 3 noodles on top followed by the spinach mixture. Spread on remaining Veggie Ground Round mixture followed by 1 cup of shredded cheese. Place the last 3 lasagna noodles on top and cover with the rest of the tomato sauce. Top lasagna with remaining shredded cheese.

Bake in the preheated oven for 45 minutes or until the noodles are tender.

Nutrition:

Calories: 529 calories

Total Fat: 20.3 g

Cholesterol: 53 mg

Sodium: 1723 mg

Total Carbohydrate: 52.4 g

Protein: 34 g

202.   Veggie Lasagna Florentine

Serving: 12
Preparation Time: 20 Minutes
Cooking Time: 1 h 25 Minutes

Ingredients

1 (16 ounce) package lasagna noodles

2 tablespoons olive oil

1 onion, chopped

1 (8 ounce) can sliced mushrooms

2 tablespoons minced garlic

1 zucchini, finely chopped

2 (28 ounce) cans crushed tomatoes

1 (6 ounce) can tomato paste

1 tablespoon dried oregano

1 pinch brown sugar

salt to taste

1 (10 ounce) package frozen chopped spinach, thawed

1 (16 ounce) container nonfat cottage cheese

2 eggs

3 tablespoons dried basil, divided

1/4 cup grated Parmesan cheese

1 pound shredded mozzarella cheese

Direction

Cook lasagna noodles in a large pot of lightly salted, boiling water for 10 minutes, or until al dente. Rinse with cool water, drain, and set aside.

Heat oil in a large skillet over medium heat. Cook the chopped onions, mushrooms, garlic, and zucchini in the oil until soft. Stir in both cans of crushed tomatoes, tomato paste, oregano, brown sugar, and salt to taste. Reduce heat to low, and simmer for 15 minutes.

Meanwhile, microwave frozen spinach until cooked. Cool, and then squeeze out excess water. Drain cottage cheese. Using a mixer, blend spinach, cottage cheese, eggs, and 2 tablespoons basil until smooth. In a separate bowl, combine shredded mozzarella cheese and grated Parmesan cheese.

Preheat oven to 350 degrees F (175 degrees C). Spread 1 cup sauce in the bottom of a 9x13 inch baking dish. Layer 1/3 of the noodles, 1/3 cottage cheese/spinach mixture, 1/3 of remaining sauce, and 1/3 cheese mixture. Repeat layers with remaining ingredients. Sprinkle top with remaining 1 tablespoon of dried basil.

Bake in preheated oven for 60 minutes. Let stand for 10 minutes before serving.

Nutrition:

Calories: 375 calories

Total Fat: 11.2 g

Cholesterol: 58 mg

Sodium: 802 mg

Total Carbohydrate: 47.3 g

Protein: 25.1 g

203. Veggie Lo Mein

Serving: 6
Preparation Time: 15 Minutes
Cooking Time: 10 Minutes

Ingredients

1 pound dry Chinese noodles

1 cup chopped fresh mushrooms

1 (8 ounce) can bamboo shoots, drained

1 cup chopped celery

1 cup bean sprouts

1/2 teaspoon chopped garlic

1 teaspoon salt

1 cup vegetable broth

1 teaspoon white sugar

1 cup water

1 tablespoon soy sauce

1 tablespoon oyster sauce

1 tablespoon all-purpose flour

Direction

Bring a large pot of lightly salted water to a boil. Add Chinese noodles and cook about 2 to 4 minutes; drain.

In a large skillet or wok over high heat with a small amount or oil, cook mushrooms, bamboo shoots, celery, bean sprouts and garlic. Mix in salt, broth, sugar, water, soy sauce and oyster sauce; stir. Add flour and cook until thickened. Pour over noodles and toss lightly.

Nutrition:

Calories: 283 calories

Total Fat: 2 g

Cholesterol: 0 mg

Sodium: 713 mg

Total Carbohydrate: 63.1 g

Protein: 10.2 g

204. Veggie Spaghetti

Serving: 6

Ingredients

1 pound spaghetti

3/4 cup margarine

1 onion, chopped

1 (28 ounce) can whole peeled tomatoes

1/2 teaspoon salt

3 tablespoons all-purpose flour

1 cup milk

1 cup heavy whipping cream

15 large black olives, halved

1 (4.5 ounce) can sliced mushrooms

1/2 cup grated Parmesan cheese

Direction

In a large skillet melt 1/2 cup margarine over medium heat. Stir in onion, chopped tomatoes, and salt; simmer for 1/2 hour.

Meanwhile, in a large pot with boiling salted water cook pasta until al dente. Drain. Place cooked spaghetti in the bottom of a greased 9x13 inch baking dish.

In a small saucepan melt 3 tablespoons of margarine over medium heat. Take off heat and quickly stir in 3 tablespoons of flour to make a paste. Return to heat and slowly stir in the milk. Cook on low, stirring often, until thick. Add heavy cream and continue to cook until slightly thickened.

Pour simmered tomato mix over top of spaghetti. Sprinkle on olive halves and mushrooms. Pour cream sauce on top. Sprinkle with grated Parmesan cheese.

Bake in a preheated 350 degree F (175 degrees C) oven for 30 minutes.

Nutrition:

Calories: 729 calories

Total Fat: 42.4 g

Cholesterol: 63 mg

Sodium: 968 mg

Total Carbohydrate: 71.7 g

Protein: 16.9 g

205.   Wendys Quick Pasta And Lentils

Serving: 6
Preparation Time: 15 Minutes
Cooking Time: 30 Minutes

Ingredients

1 onion, chopped

3 cloves garlic, minced

2 tablespoons olive oil

1 (19 ounce) can lentil soup

1 cup crushed tomatoes

1 (10 ounce) package frozen chopped spinach

1 (16 ounce) package ditalini pasta

salt to taste

ground black pepper to taste

1 pinch crushed red pepper

2 tablespoons grated Parmesan cheese

Direction

Brown onion and garlic in oil over medium heat. Stir in lentil soup and tomatoes. Bring to boil. Stir in spinach and spices. Simmer.

Meanwhile, cook pasta in a large pot of boiling salted water until almost done. Drain. Mix pasta into lentil sauce. Cover, and keep warm for 20 minutes. Serve with Parmesan cheese.

Nutrition:

Calories: 407 calories

Total Fat: 7.1 g

Cholesterol: 1 mg

Sodium: 282 mg

Total Carbohydrate: 70.5 g

Protein: 15.9 g

206.   Ziti And Eggplant

Serving: 6
Preparation Time: 15 Minutes
Cooking Time: 1 hours

Ingredients

2 tablespoons olive oil

1 eggplant, peeled and cut into 1/2-inch cubes

1 (28 ounce) can crushed tomatoes

2 tablespoons minced fresh basil

ground black pepper to taste

1 1/4 teaspoons white sugar (optional)

1 (7 ounce) jar roasted red pepper, drained and cut into strips

1 (16 ounce) package dry ziti pasta

3 pita bread rounds

2 tablespoons butter

1/4 cup grated Parmesan cheese or to taste

sweet paprika to taste

salt and pepper to taste

Direction

Heat the olive oil in a skillet over medium heat, and cook the eggplant about 10 minutes. Stir in the tomatoes, basil, pepper, and sugar. Simmer, stirring occasionally, 45 minutes. Mix the roasted red peppers into the skillet with the eggplant mixture. Continue cooking until eggplant is the consistency of the rest of the sauce.

Bring a large pot of lightly salted water to a boil. Place ziti pasta in the pot, cook 9 to 11 minutes, until al dente, and drain. Serve the eggplant and tomato sauce over the cooked ziti.

Preheat oven to 375 degrees F (190 degrees C). Open pitas and evenly spread insides with butter. Sprinkle with Parmesan cheese and season with paprika, salt and pepper. I like to make a light sprinkling of paprika across each piece. Heat pitas in the preheated oven until golden brown, about 6 minutes. Use to scoop up eggplant sauce, or eat separately.

Nutrition:

Calories: 545 calories

Total Fat: 12.1 g

Cholesterol: 13 mg

Sodium: 534 mg

Total Carbohydrate: 91.9 g

Protein: 18.4 g

207.   Ziti With Tomato Pesto Sauce

Serving: 6
Preparation Time: 5 Minutes
Cooking Time: 20 Minutes

Ingredients

12 ounces ziti pasta

2 tablespoons pesto

1 (26 ounce) jar tomato basil pasta sauce

salt to taste

1/2 cup grated Parmesan cheese

Direction

Bring a large pot of lightly salted water to a boil. Add ziti pasta, and cook until al dente, about 8 minutes. Drain.

Meanwhile, in a saucepan over medium-low heat, mix together the pesto and basil tomato sauce. Bring to a simmer, and season with salt to taste. (You can also heat the sauce in a covered microwave-safe bowl: cook on high for one minute.)

Place pasta in a large serving bowl. Toss with pesto-tomato sauce. Top with grated Parmesan cheese.

Nutrition:

Calories: 368 calories

Total Fat: 8.4 g

Cholesterol: 10 mg

Sodium: 642 mg

Total Carbohydrate: 59.1 g

Protein: 13 g

208.   Zoodle Lasagne

Serving: 4
Preparation Time: 20 Minutes
Cooking Time: 35 Minutes

Ingredients

4 zucchini

1 1/2 cups homemade or store-bought tomato sauce

2/3 cup shredded mozzarella cheese

1 1/2 cups bechamel sauce

1 cup grated Parmigiano Reggiano cheese

1/4 cup fresh basil, chopped

Direction

Preheat oven to 375 degrees F (190 degrees C).

Cut zucchini lengthwise into 1/4-inch thick slices with a knife or mandolin.

Pour 2 tablespoons tomato sauce on the bottom of a 9x13-inch baking dish. Arrange zucchini slices in a single layer, slightly overlapping, over tomato sauce.

Top with a thin layer of mozzarella, 1/3 of the bechamel (see Editor's Note), 1/3 of remaining tomato sauce, 1/3 of the Parmigiano Reggiano cheese, and 1/3 of the basil. Repeat layers, topping with bechamel and Parmigiano Reggiano cheese.

Bake in the preheated oven until sauce is bubbly and the top is golden brown, about 35 minutes. Allow to set until remaining liquid is absorbed, about 10 minutes.

Nutrition:

Calories: 281 calories

Total Fat: 18.1 g

Cholesterol: 53 mg

Sodium: 1778 mg

Total Carbohydrate: 15.5 g

Protein: 16.2 g

209.   Zucchini And Shells

Serving: 4
Preparation Time: 15 Minutes
Cooking Time: 1 hours

Ingredients

1/4 cup olive oil

1/2 medium onion, finely chopped

3 cloves garlic, minced

1 large zucchini, peeled and cubed

1 (15 ounce) can tomato sauce

2 cups water

1 teaspoon dried oregano

1 teaspoon dried basil

1/8 teaspoon crushed red pepper flakes

1/2 cup white sugar

1 (8 ounce) package uncooked pasta shells

1/4 cup grated Romano cheese

Direction

Heat the olive oil in a saucepan over medium heat. Stir in the onion and garlic, and cook until tender. Mix in zucchini and coat in the olive oil. Pour in tomato sauce and water. Season with oregano, basil, and red pepper. Dissolve sugar in the sauce. Reduce heat to low, and simmer 1 hour, stirring occasionally.

Bring a large pot of lightly salted water to a boil. Add pasta and cook for 8 to 10 minutes or until al dente; drain.

In a large bowl, mix sauce and cooked pasta shells. Top with cheese to serve.

Nutrition:

Calories: 515 calories

Total Fat: 17.2 g

Cholesterol: 8 mg

Sodium: 650 mg

Total Carbohydrate: 79.3 g

Protein: 13.3 g

210.   Zucchini Linguine

Serving: 4
Preparation Time: 15 Minutes
Cooking Time: 15 Minutes

Ingredients

1 (8 ounce) package linguine pasta

1 tablespoon olive oil

2 cloves garlic, minced

3 zucchini, shredded

1/4 cup shredded Cheddar cheese

1/4 cup plain nonfat yogurt

salt and pepper to taste

Direction

Bring a large pot of lightly salted water to a boil. Add pasta and cook for 8 to 10 minutes or until al dente; drain.

Meanwhile, heat oil in a large skillet over medium heat. Sauté garlic until it starts to brown. Stir in a handful of grated zucchini; cook for 1 minute and then add the rest of the zucchini. Cook for 3 minutes.

Toss pasta with zucchini, cheese and yogurt. Season with salt and pepper. Mix well and serve.

Nutrition:

Calories: 290 calories

Total Fat: 7.2 g

Cholesterol: 8 mg

Sodium: 63 mg

Total Carbohydrate: 46.8 g

Protein: 11.9 g

211.   Zucchini Pasta

Serving: 8

Ingredients

1 pound rotini pasta

5 small zucchini, sliced

1/3 cup olive oil

4 cloves garlic, minced

1 pinch crushed red pepper flakes

1/3 cup chopped fresh parsley

salt and pepper to taste

1/2 cup grated Parmesan cheese

Direction

Bring a large pot of lightly salted water to a boil. Add pasta and cook for 8 to 10 minutes or until al dente. Drain and reserve.

Fill a medium sauce pan with lightly salted water. Add zucchini and bring to a boil; boil for 10 minutes or until tender.

In a large skillet, sauté garlic in oil and hot pepper flakes. Add drained zucchini and parsley, then mix all together and simmer for 5 to 10 minutes. Toss with pasta; then add cheese and salt and pepper to taste, and serve.

Nutrition:

Calories: 320 calories

Total Fat: 11.9 g

Cholesterol: 4 mg

Sodium: 89 mg

Total Carbohydrate: 44.7 g

Protein: 10.5 g

212.   Zucchini Pasta Bake

Serving: 6
Preparation Time: 15 Minutes
Cooking Time: 25 Minutes

Ingredients

8 ounces penne pasta

1/4 cup Parmesan cheese

1/2 cup crushed saltine crackers

1 tablespoon olive oil

1/2 onion, chopped

2 cups chopped zucchini

1 tomato, chopped

2 cloves garlic, minced

1/2 teaspoon dried oregano

1/2 teaspoon dried basil

1 pinch dried celery flakes

salt and pepper to taste

1 cup shredded mozzarella cheese

Direction

Bring a large pot of lightly salted water to a boil. Add penne pasta, cook for 10 to 12 minutes, until al dente, and drain. Lightly grease a medium casserole dish.

Preheat oven to 350 degrees F (175 degrees C). In a blender or food processor, thoroughly mix the Parmesan cheese and crackers.

Heat the oil in a skillet over medium heat. Place the onion in the skillet, and cook and stir until tender. Mix in the zucchini, tomato, and garlic, and season with oregano, basil, celery, salt, and pepper. Continue to cook and stir until the zucchini is tender.

In the prepared casserole dish, mix the pasta with the vegetable mixture and mozzarella cheese. Top evenly with the Parmesan cheese mixture.

Bake 25 minutes in the preheated oven, or until the topping is lightly browned. Allow to sit 5 minutes before serving.

Nutrition:

Calories: 271 calories

Total Fat: 7.9 g

Cholesterol: 15 mg

Sodium: 336 mg

Total Carbohydrate: 37.2 g

Protein: 12.7 g

213. Zucchini With Mushroom Ravioli In Truffle Butter Sauce

Serving: 2
Preparation Time: 10 Minutes
Cooking Time: 20 Minutes

Ingredients

1 tablespoon butter

3 cloves garlic, minced

3 zucchinis, sliced

1 (9 ounce) package mushroom ravioli

salt and ground black pepper to taste

1 tablespoon butter

1 teaspoon white truffle oil

Direction

Bring a pot of salted water to a boil. While water is heating, melt 1 tablespoon of butter in a large skillet over medium heat, and cook the garlic until fragrant but not brown, about 1 minute. Stir in the zucchini slices, and cook until tender and slightly browned, about 10 minutes. Season to taste with salt and pepper.

About 5 minutes after starting to cook the zucchini, stir the mushroom ravioli into the boiling water. Let them cook until they begin to float, about 5 minutes; scoop out the ravioli with a slotted spoon, and add them to the zucchini. Melt 1 more tablespoon of butter with the ravioli and zucchini, and drizzle the dish with truffle oil. Gently toss the ravioli and zucchini to thoroughly coat with butter and truffle oil, and serve.

Nutrition:

Calories: 410 calories

Total Fat: 19.6 g

Cholesterol: 71 mg

Sodium: 370 mg

Total Carbohydrate: 47 g

Protein: 13.3 g

214.   Pink Pasta

Serving: 4
Preparation Time: 10 Minutes
Cooking Time: 20 Minutes

Ingredients

1 (8 ounce) package campanelle (little bells) pasta

1/2 cup ricotta cheese

2 tablespoons olive oil

1/4 onion, chopped

1 (6.5 ounce) can tomato sauce

1/4 cup chopped fresh basil

1 tablespoon chopped fresh oregano

Direction

Bring a large pot of lightly salted water to a boil. Cook the campanelle pasta at a boil, stirring occasionally, until cooked through yet firm to the bite, about 12 minutes; drain. Transfer pasta to a large bowl, add ricotta cheese, and stir so the ricotta begins to melt into the pasta.

Heat olive oil in a large skillet over medium-high heat. Sauté onion in olive oil until lightly browned, 5 to 7 minutes. Sir tomato sauce, basil, and oregano with the onion; bring to a simmer and cook another 2 to 3 minutes.

Pour tomato sauce over the pasta and stir until the sauce and cheese evenly coat the pasta.

Nutrition:

Calories: 328 calories

Total Fat: 10.2 g

Cholesterol: 10 mg

Sodium: 284 mg

Total Carbohydrate: 47.4 g

Protein: 11.7 g

215.   Polish Cabbage Noodles

Serving: 5

Ingredients

1 medium head shredded cabbage

2 red onions, cut into strips

1/2 cup butter

1 (16 ounce) package wide egg noodles

salt to taste

ground black pepper to taste

Direction

Cook pasta in a large pot of boiling salted water.

Meanwhile, heat butter or margarine in a skillet over medium heat. Sauté cabbage and onions until tender.

Drain pasta, and return to the pot. Add cabbage and onion mixture to the noodles, and toss. Season with salt and pepper to taste.

Nutrition:

Calories: 570 calories

Total Fat: 22.6 g

Cholesterol: 124 mg

Sodium: 184 mg

Total Carbohydrate: 78.5 g

Protein: 15.7 g

216. Polish Style Lasagna

Serving: 6
Preparation Time: 20 Minutes
Cooking Time: 20 Minutes

Ingredients

9 uncooked lasagna noodles

1 onion, sliced

1/2 cup butter

2 2/3 cups dry potato flakes

1 (8 ounce) package cream cheese

Direction

Preheat oven to 350 degrees F (175 degrees C).

Cook lasagna noodles according to package directions. Drain, pat dry and interleave in a damp towel to keep moist OR spray each noodle with cooking spray OR lightly apply some oil.

In a separate large skillet over medium heat, combine the onions with the butter and sauté for 5 minutes.

Prepare the instant mashed potatoes according to package directions, but omit the milk. Stir in the cream cheese until well blended.

Place 3 noodles in the bottom of a lightly greased 9x13-inch baking dish. Spread 1/2 the potato mixture over the noodles in the dish. Top this with 3 more noodles, followed by the other 1/2 of the potato mixture. Finish by topping with the remaining 3 noodles, then top those with sautéed onions.

Bake at 350 degrees F (175 degrees C) for 20 minutes, or until bubbly. Allow to cool for 5 minutes before cutting.

Nutrition:

Calories: 415 calories

Total Fat: 29.3 g

Cholesterol: 83 mg

Sodium: 246 mg

Total Carbohydrate: 32.5 g

Protein: 7.3 g

217.   Porcini Mushroom Pasta

Serving: 6

Ingredients

1 tablespoon olive oil

2 cloves garlic, minced

1/2 red onion, minced

1/2 cup red bell pepper, julienned

1/2 cup julienned carrots

1/2 cup dry red wine

1 cup rehydrated porcini mushrooms

1 1/2 cups crushed tomatoes

2 teaspoons chopped fresh basil

1 teaspoon dried rosemary, crushed

salt and pepper to taste

6 cups tagliatelle (wide noodles)

Direction

Heat the oil in a large skillet over medium heat. Add garlic and onions and sauté for 4 minutes, then add red bell pepper and carrots and sauté for 4 more minutes. Add red wine, raise heat and boil for 1 minute; then reduce heat to medium low, add mushrooms and cook for 3 minutes.

Add tomatoes, basil and rosemary and season with salt and pepper to taste. Simmer for 10 minutes and serve sauce over cooked noodles.

Nutrition:

Calories: 335 calories

Total Fat: 4.3 g

Cholesterol: 0 mg

Sodium: 19 mg

Total Carbohydrate: 56.1 g

Protein: 13.8 g

218.   Portobello Bellybuttons

Serving: 4
Preparation Time: 15 Minutes
Cooking Time: 15 Minutes

Ingredients

1 (16 ounce) package cheese tortellini

3 tablespoons butter

1 clove garlic, minced

2 portobello mushrooms, chopped

1/2 pound button mushrooms, sliced

1/4 cup white wine

1/2 tablespoon dried basil

salt and pepper to taste

1/2 cup grated Parmesan cheese

Direction

Bring a large pot of lightly salted water to a boil. Add pasta and cook until al dente; drain.

While water is boiling, melt the butter in a skillet and cook the garlic until fragrant. Stir in portobello mushrooms, button mushrooms, white wine, and basil. Season with salt and pepper to taste. Continue to cook until mushrooms are tender. Pour mushroom mixture into drained pasta and stir. Top with grated Parmesan cheese and serve.

Nutrition:

Calories: 512 calories

Total Fat: 21.6 g

Cholesterol: 81 mg

Sodium: 778 mg

Total Carbohydrate: 57.8 g

Protein: 22.6 g

219.   Portobello Mushroom Stroganoff

Serving: 4
Preparation Time: 10 Minutes
Cooking Time: 20 Minutes

Ingredients

3 tablespoons butter

1 large onion, chopped

3/4 pound portobello mushrooms, sliced

1 1/2 cups vegetable broth

1 1/2 cups sour cream

3 tablespoons all-purpose flour

1/4 cup chopped fresh parsley

8 ounces dried egg noodles

Direction

Bring a large pot of lightly salted water to a boil. Add egg noodles, and cook until al dente, about 7 minutes. Remove from heat, drain, and set aside.

At the same time, melt butter in a large heavy skillet over medium heat. Add onion, and cook, stirring until softened. Turn the heat up to medium-high, and add sliced mushrooms. Cook until the mushrooms are limp and browned. Remove to a bowl, and set aside.

In the same skillet, stir in vegetable broth, being sure to stir in any browned bits off the bottom of the pan. Bring to a boil, and cook until the mixture has reduced by 1/3. Reduce heat to low, and return the mushrooms and onion to the skillet.

Remove the pan from the heat, stir together the sour cream and flour; then blend into the mushrooms. Return the skillet to the burner, and continue cooking over low heat, just until the sauce thickens. Stir in the parsley, and season to taste with salt and pepper. Serve over cooked egg noodles.

Nutrition:

Calories: 525 calories

Total Fat: 30.1 g

Cholesterol: 101 mg

Sodium: 295 mg

Total Carbohydrate: 53.3 g

Protein: 12.8 g

220.   Vermicelli Salad With Crabmeat

8 oz. vermicelli

8 black Chinese dried mushrooms

1 lb. crabmeat

4 scallions, sliced

1 cup water chestnuts, drained and cut into thin strips

1 cup bamboo shoots, drained and cut into thin strips

2 tablespoons soy sauce

2 tablespoons sweet and sour sauce

3 drops hot chili sauce

3 tablespoons oil

3 tablespoons lemon juice

Cook pasta according to package directions until al dente; drain.

Place mushrooms in bowl and cover with boiling water; let soak for 30 minutes. Drain and cut into strips.

In a large bowl, combine pasta, mushrooms, crabmeat, scallions, water chestnuts, bamboo shoots, soy sauce, sweet and sour sauce, chili sauce, and oil; mix well. Sprinkle salad with lemon juice, and serve.

Yield: 4

221.   Light And Easy Pasta Salad

2 cups (8 oz.) rotini pasta

2/3 cup reduced calorie Italian dressing

1 cup halved cherry tomatoes

2 cups halved zucchini slices

1 cup sliced mushrooms

1 cup (4 oz.) reduced fat Cheddar cheese, shredded

2 tablespoons Parmesan cheese

Cook pasta according to package directions; drain.

Mix Italian dressing with tomatoes, zucchini, mushrooms and pasta; cover. Chill several hours. Toss with Cheddar cheese. Serve on a lettuce leaf-lined platter and sprinkle with Parmesan cheese.

Yield: 6

222. Pizza Salad

8 oz. rotini

1 lb. diced cheese, mild or sharp Cheddar

3 tomatoes, chopped, seeded

1 to 2 bunches scallions, sliced

3 oz. pepperoni, sliced

Dressing:

3/4 cup olive oil

1/2 cup red wine vinegar (or white vinegar)

2/3 cup Parmesan cheese

2 teaspoons dried oregano

1 teaspoon garlic powder

Salt and pepper

Croutons

Cook pasta according to package directions; drain. In a large bowl, combine rotini, cheese, tomatoes, scallions and pepperoni.

Mix oil with vinegar, Parmesan cheese, oregano, garlic powder, salt and pepper; pour over pasta mixture. Chill 4 hours; Toss and garnish with croutons.

Yield: 4

223.   Fire And Ice Pasta Salad

1 lb. rotini or spaghetti

1/2 cup olive oil

1/4 teaspoon chili flakes

1 garlic clove, crushed, minced

1 teaspoon salt

1/4 teaspoon pepper

2 lb. tomatoes (about 6), diced

1/4 cup chopped fresh basil

1/4 cup chopped fresh parsley

2 tablespoons chopped fresh chives

Cook pasta according to package directions; drain.

Blend olive oil with chili flakes, garlic, salt and pepper. Mix with tomatoes, basil, parsley and chives. Let stand at room temperature, covered, for 20 minutes to 1 hour. Toss with pasta and serve.

Yield: 4 to 6

224.   Best Pasta Salad

8 oz. rotini pasta

1 large tomato, chopped

1 medium red bell pepper, chopped

1 can black olives, sliced

1 medium green bell pepper, chopped

1 small onion, chopped

1/4 cup Parmesan cheese

1 (8 oz.) bottle sun dried tomato vinaigrette dressing

Cook pasta according to package directions; drain and rinse in cold water.

Mix tomato, bell pepper, olives, bell pepper and onion. Add pasta and chill one hour; mix with salad dressing. Toss with Parmesan cheese.

Yield: 4

225.   Greek Rotini Salad

1 (12 oz.) pkg. rotini, tricolor

1 cup feta cheese, Roquefort or blue cheese, crumbled

1/2 cup black olives, coarsely chopped

3/4 cup radishes, sliced

1/4 cup green onion, sliced

1 small cucumber, thinly sliced

Dressing:

1/2 cup olive oil or vegetable oil

2 tablespoons lemon juice

2 tablespoons fresh parsley, chopped

1 clove garlic, minced

1 teaspoon Italian seasoning

1 teaspoon lemon pepper, or lemon and herb seasoning

1 teaspoon basil

Cook pasta according to package directions; drain. In a large bowl, toss hot cooked rotini with cheese, olives, radishes, onions and cucumber.

In a small bowl, combine oil with lemon juice, parsley, garlic, Italian seasoning, lemon pepper and basil; toss with pasta mix and add salt and pepper as needed. Refrigerate 1 to 2 hours before serving.

Yield: 6 to 8

226.   Penne Pasta Salad

1 lb. penne pasta

1 red bell pepper, julienned

1 bunch scallions or green onions

1 bunch asparagus, cooked, chopped in 1-inch pieces

1 (13.75) can artichoke hearts

1/4 cup olive oil

10 sun-dried tomatoes, chopped

8 oz. feta cheese, cubed

1 (8 oz.) bottle vinaigrette salad dressing

2 cloves garlic, chopped

2 tablespoons pesto (optional)

Cook pasta according to package directions; drain. Sauté bell pepper in a little olive oil. Mix all ingredients and chill in covered container. Toss before serving.

Yield: 6 - 8

227. Piquant Vermicelli

8 oz. vermicelli

1/4 cup butter

1/4 lb. mushrooms, thinly sliced

1 teaspoon marjoram

2 tablespoons chopped parsley

Salt and pepper to taste

Cook pasta according to package directions; drain. Place in serving bowl and keep warm.

Melt butter in a small saucepan. Add mushrooms; cook over low heat stirring constantly for 3 minutes. Spoon mushrooms over vermicelli. Add marjoram, parsley, salt and pepper; toss until well mixed. Serve at once.

Yield: 6

228.   Rigatoni Salad

1 (16 oz. pkg.) rigatoni

1 cup granulated sugar

1 teaspoon salt

1 teaspoon Accent

1 teaspoon garlic powder

1 cup vegetable oil

1 cup vinegar

1 teaspoon pepper

1 teaspoon parsley flakes

1 cucumber, diced

1 medium onion, diced

Cook pasta according to directions on package; drain.

In a medium bowl, combine sugar, salt, Accent, garlic powder, vegetable oil, vinegar, pepper and parsley.

Combine seasoned oil with pasta, onion and cucumber. Refrigerate at least 48 hours. Stir occasionally.

Yield: 6 to 8

229.   Cashew Tortellini Chicken Salad

2 cups cheese tortellini

2 cups frozen sugar snap peas

2 cups cooked chicken, diced

1/4 cup celery, chopped

3 tablespoons green onions, sliced

1 tablespoon pimientos, chopped

1/4 teaspoon salt

1/2 cup reduced fat ranch dressing

1/4 cup whole cashews

Leaf lettuce

Cook pasta according to directions on package; drain and rinse with cold water.

Thaw sugar snap peas in water; drain. In a large bowl, combine chicken, celery, green onions, pimientos, salt and snap peas. Pour dressing over salad; mix to coat. Refrigerate at least 2 to 3 hours. Serve on lettuce leaf and garnish with cashews.

Yield: 2

230. Shrimp Salad

1 (7 oz.) pkg. elbow macaroni

2 hard cooked eggs, chopped

1 cup celery, chopped

2 (4 oz. each) cans shrimp

1/8 cup green bell pepper, chopped

1 green onion, sliced

1 tablespoon pimento

Dressing:

1 cup salad dressing or mayonnaise

3 tablespoons cream

Cook pasta according to directions on package; rinse, drain and cool.

In a large bowl, mix macaroni, eggs, celery, shrimp, bell pepper, onion and pimento. Add dressing and toss to coat evenly.

Yield: 12

231.   Green Tomato Pasta

4 cups spaghetti

4 large green tomatoes, thinly sliced (1/8-inch thick)

Salt and pepper, to taste

1 cup flour

Vegetable oil, for frying

2 garlic cloves, minced

1/4 cup parmesan cheese, grated

Prepare spaghetti according to package directions; drain well and set aside.

Season tomatoes with salt and pepper. Coat with flour and fry in hot oil with garlic until golden brown. Do not overcook. Place fried tomato slices on top of hot, cooked pasta. Top with parmesan cheese and serve immediately.

Yield: 4

232.   Ham, Peas And Cheese Salad

1 (7 oz.) pkg. elbow macaroni

1 (10 oz.) pkg. frozen peas

1 cup cheddar cheese, cubed

2 cups cooked ham, cubed

1 cup salad dressing (not mayonnaise)

2 tablespoons onions, minced

3/4 teaspoon salt

1/4 teaspoon pepper

1 teaspoon lemon juice

Cook pasta according to directions on package; rinse, drain and cool.

Cover peas with boiling water, but do not cook. Let peas stand in hot water 5 minutes; drain. Mix macaroni and peas, cheese and ham.

In a small bowl, blend dressing, onion, salt, pepper and lemon juice. Pour dressing over macaroni mix and toss gently to coat. Refrigerate at least one hour.

Yield: 4

233.   Shrimp Salad

Mix together:

1 (7 oz.) pkg. medium shell pasta (cooked, rinsed and drained)

1 (12 oz.) pkg. little frozen shrimp

1 cup celery, chopped

3/4 cup frozen peas

Diced cheese

Set aside.

Dressing:

1/3 cup granulated sugar

1/3 cup vegetable oil

1 cup mayonnaise

1/4 cup ketchup

1/4 cup vinegar

1 teaspoon dry mustard

1/4 teaspoon paprika

1 medium onion, chopped

1/4 teaspoon salt

Garlic salt and pepper to taste

In a small bowl, mix dressing ingredients and toss with macaroni mixture. Add garlic salt and pepper to taste. Dressing is thin, but it thickens when chilled.

Yield: 4

234.   Armenian Pilaf

6 tablespoons butter or margarine

1 1/2 cups broken pieces vermicelli

1 cup rice

1/2 teaspoon salt

2 cups boiling water

In a large saucepan, melt butter or margarine; add vermicelli. Cook over medium-high heat, stirring until well browned. Add rice, salt and boiling water; stir and cover. Boil slowly for 10 minutes.

Remove from heat and let stand covered for 15 to 20 minutes. Keep warm in oven if not served immediately.

Yield: 6

235.   Ham And Macaroni Salad

2 cups elbow macaroni

1/2 lb. boiled or baked ham, diced

1/2 cup cheddar cheese, diced

1 small onion, chopped

1 cup celery, chopped

1/2 cup dill pickle, diced

1/2 cup mayonnaise

2 teaspoons prepared mustard

Lettuce leaves

3 to 6 hard-boiled eggs, sliced

3 tomatoes, quartered

Cook pasta according to directions on package; drain. In a medium bowl, combine ham, cheese, onion, celery and pickles with macaroni.

Mix mayonnaise with mustard and stir into macaroni mixture; chill until ready to serve. Serve spooned onto lettuce leaves and garnished with eggs and tomatoes.

Yield: 6

236.   Acini De Pepe Pasta Fruit Salad

1 cup granulated sugar

2 tablespoons flour

1/2 teaspoon salt

1 3/4 cups pineapple juice

2 eggs, beaten

1 tablespoon lemon juice

1 (16 oz.) pkg. acini de pepe pasta

3 (11 oz. each) cans mandarin oranges, drained

2 (20 oz. each) cans pineapple chunks, drained

1 (20 oz.) can crushed pineapple, drained

1 (8 oz.) tub Cool Whip

1 cup flaked coconut, optional

2 cups miniature marshmallows, optional

Combine sugar, flour and salt in a small saucepan. Stir in pineapple juice and eggs. Stirring constantly, simmer over moderate heat until thickened. Blend in lemon juice; cool sauce to room temperature.

Cook pasta according to directions on package; drain, rinse in cold water, drain again. Gently blend egg mix and macaroni. Refrigerate overnight in sealed container.

The next morning, add fruit, Cool Whip, coconut and marshmallows. Fold gently to incorporate ingredients. Refrigerate in sealed container until chilled. Prepare 24 hours before serving.

Note: Fresh fruit can be substituted for canned.

Yield: 25

237.   Macaroni Fruit Salad

1/2 pkg. elbow macaroni

1 large apple, diced

1/2 jar maraschino cherries and juice, quartered

1/2 pkg. small marshmallows

1/2 cup crushed pineapple with juice

1/2 cup granulated sugar or sugar substitute

1/2 cup lemon juice

2 eggs, beaten

1 tablespoon flour

1/2 pint fat free nondairy whipped topping

Cook pasta according to package directions; rinse, drain and cool. Combine apple, macaroni, cherries, marshmallows and pineapple in a large bowl.

In a small saucepan, mix sugar, lemon juice, eggs and flour, cooking and stirring until bubbling; cool and mix into salad. Refrigerate overnight. Before serving, add 1/2 pint nondairy whipped topping to salad.

Yield: 3 to 4

238.   Italian Pasta Salad

1 lb. small shell pasta

4 oz. provolone cheese, chopped

4 oz. salami, chopped

4 oz. pepperoni, chopped

2 small onions, chopped

1/2 cup celery, chopped

1/2 cup green bell pepper, chopped

1/2 cup red bell pepper, chopped

1 (2.25) can pitted black olives, chopped

1 (7 oz.) jar green olives, chopped

3 to 5 ripe tomatoes, chopped

Fresh parsley to taste

Dressing:

3/4 cup olive oil

1/2 cup white vinegar

1 tablespoon salt

1 teaspoon pepper

3 tablespoons granulated sugar

1 tablespoon oregano

Cook pasta according to package directions; drain. In a large bowl, combine with cheese, salami, pepperoni, onions, celery, green bell pepper, red bell pepper, black olives and green olives.

In a small bowl, combine olive oil, vinegar, sugar, oregano, salt and pepper. Gently toss with salad and chill for 24 hours. Add the tomatoes and parsley just before serving.

Yield: 15

239. Macaroni And Chicken Salad

1 (16 oz.) pkg. elbow macaroni

1/2 cup reduced fat French dressing

1 1/3 cups reduced fat mayonnaise

1 chicken, cooked and cut into bite-size pieces

1 teaspoon salt

1/2 green bell pepper, chopped

2 cups celery, sliced

2/3 cup sweet pickle relish

2 tablespoons onions, minced

Cook pasta according to package directions; drain and cool. Blend French dressing with mayonnaise; mix in chicken, salt, bell pepper, celery, relish and onion. Mix with macaroni. Chill.

Yield: 8

240. Hearty Macaroni Salad

2 cups ham, cubed

2 cups cooked chicken, cubed

2 cups cooked salad shrimp

1 (7 oz.) pkg. elbow macaroni

2 cups celery, chopped

1/4 cup green bell pepper, diced

1/4 cup sweet red bell pepper, diced

1/2 cup onion diced

1 teaspoon salt

1/2 teaspoon pepper

Toss all ingredients together in a large bowl.

Dressing:

1/2 cup light mayonnaise

1/2 cup reduced fat sour cream

2 teaspoons vinegar

1/2 teaspoon granulated sugar

2 teaspoons fresh dill, minced

In a small bowl, mix dressing ingredients; pour on salad and gently toss to blend. Cover. Chill 3 to 4 hours.

Yield: 12

241. Spring Salad With Shell Pasta

1 (16 oz.) pkg. small shell pasta

1 large cucumber, diced

1 onion, chopped fine

3 medium carrots, grated

3 ribs celery, sliced thin

1 green bell pepper, chopped

Dressing:

2 cups reduced fat mayonnaise

1 cup granulated sugar

1 cup white vinegar

1 (14 oz.) can fat free sweetened condensed milk

Cook pasta according to package directions; drain. Combine pasta with vegetables in a large bowl. Pour dressing over ingredients and toss to coat.

Yield: 12 to 15

242.   Smoked Turkey And Pepper Pasta Salad

8 oz. fettuccine

3/4 cup reduced fat Miracle Whip

1 tablespoon Dijon mustard

1/2 teaspoon dried thyme

1 cup (8 oz.) smoked turkey breast, diced

3/4 cup zucchini slices, halved

1/2 cup red bell pepper strips

1/2 cup yellow bell pepper strips

Salt and pepper to taste

Cook fettuccine according to package directions; drain and rinse.

Mix salad dressing, mustard and thyme until well blended. Add pasta, turkey, zucchini, red and yellow bell pepper strips; mix lightly. Season with salt and pepper to taste. Chill for 4 hours.

Yield: 4

243.   Potato And Cheese Filling For Pierogi

Serving: 6

Ingredients

4 pounds mashed potatoes

1 pound shredded Cheddar cheese

salt and pepper to taste

Direction

In a large bowl, mix together mashed potatoes and shredded Cheddar cheese. Season with salt and pepper to taste.

Nutrition:

Calories: 538 calories

Total Fat: 25.3 g

Cholesterol: 79 mg

Sodium: 488 mg

Total Carbohydrate: 53.8 g

Protein: 25 g

244.   Potato Lasagna

Serving: 4
Preparation Time: 15 Minutes
Cooking Time: 45 Minutes

Ingredients
10 small red potatoes, thinly sliced
10 baby carrots, sliced
1 large green bell pepper, chopped
1/2 Vidalia onion, chopped
3 cloves garlic, chopped
2 cups baby spinach leaves
1/4 cup shredded smoked Gouda cheese
1 1/2 cups shredded mozzarella cheese
1/2 cup shredded sharp Cheddar cheese
salt and pepper to taste
1 (14 ounce) jar vodka marinara sauce
Direction
Preheat the oven to 350 degrees F (175 degrees C). Lightly grease a 2 quart
casserole dish.

In a medium bowl, toss together the carrots, bell pepper, onion, garlic, and
spinach. In a separate bowl, blend together the Gouda cheese, mozzarella
cheese, and sharp Cheddar cheese. Set aside.

Place two layers of sliced potatoes in the bottom of the prepared casserole
dish. Season the potatoes with a little salt and pepper. Top with a layer of
the spinach mixture, and pour about 1/2 cup of sauce over all. Sprinkle with
some of the cheese blend. Repeat layering with remaining potatoes,
vegetables, sauce and cheese, ending with cheese on the top.

Bake covered for 35 minutes in the preheated oven. Remove the lid, and
bake for 10 more minutes until the top is browned.

Nutrition:
Calories: 642 calories
Total Fat: 16.7 g
Cholesterol: 52 mg
Sodium: 862 mg
Total Carbohydrate: 99.4 g
Protein: 25.8 g

245.   Pumpkin Lasagna

Serving: 10
Preparation Time: 35 Minutes
Cooking Time: 40 Minutes

Ingredients

1 tablespoon minced fresh sage, divided

2 teaspoons salt, divided

1 teaspoon ground black pepper, divided

1/2 teaspoon ground nutmeg

1/2 teaspoon ground cloves

2 tablespoons olive oil

1 1/2 pounds sliced baby bella mushrooms

1 large onion, diced

2 cloves garlic, minced

3 cups pumpkin puree, divided

1 1/2 cups heavy whipping cream, divided

1 1/2 cups grated Parmesan cheese

cooking spray

12 lasagna noodles

1 cup ricotta cheese

1 cup shredded mozzarella cheese

1 dash ground nutmeg

1 dash ground cloves

2 tablespoons butter, cut in small pieces

Direction

Preheat oven to 400 degrees F (200 degrees C).

Mix sage, salt, black pepper, 1/2 teaspoon nutmeg, and 1/2 teaspoon cloves together in a small bowl to make a spice blend.

Heat olive oil in a large skillet over medium-high heat. Add mushrooms, onion, garlic, and 1/2 of the spice blend; cook and stir until mushrooms are tender and all moisture has evaporated, about 5 minutes.

Combine 2 cups pumpkin puree, 3/4 cup heavy cream, 1/2 cup Parmesan cheese, and remaining spice blend in a bowl.

Grease a 9x13-inch baking pan with cooking spray. Arrange 4 lasagna noodles in the bottom so they slightly overlap. Cover with 1/2 of the pumpkin mixture and 1/2 of the mushroom mixture. Dot with 1/2 cup ricotta; sprinkle 1/2 cup mozzarella cheese on top. Repeat layers once more. Place remaining 4 noodles on top.

Combine remaining 1 cup pumpkin puree, remaining 3/4 cup heavy cream, 1 dash nutmeg, and 1 dash cloves. Spread on top of noodles. Sprinkle remaining 1 cup Parmesan cheese on top. Dot with butter. Cover with aluminum foil.

Bake in the preheated oven for 20 minutes. Uncover and bake until bubbly, about 15 minutes more.

Nutrition:

Calories: 401 calories

Total Fat: 24.7 g

Cholesterol: 73 mg

Sodium: 932 mg

Total Carbohydrate: 33 g

Protein: 15.1 g

246. Pumpkin Ravioli

Serving: 6

Ingredients

1 cup ricotta cheese

1/2 cup pumpkin puree

1/2 teaspoon salt

1/4 teaspoon ground nutmeg

2 cups all-purpose flour

1/2 teaspoon salt

1/4 cup tomato paste

1 tablespoon olive oil

2 eggs

2 tablespoons water

Direction

Mix the cheese, pumpkin, 1/2 teaspoon salt, and the nutmeg. Set filling aside.

Mix the flour, and 1/2 teaspoon salt in a large bowl; make a well in the center of the flour. Beat the tomato paste, oil, and eggs until well blended, and pour into the well in the flour. Stir with a fork, gradually bring the flour mixture to the center of the bow until the dough makes a ball. If the dough is too dry, mix in up to 2 tablespoons water.

Knead lightly on a floured cloth-covered surface, adding flour if dough is sticky, until smooth and elastic, about 5 minutes. Cover, and let rest for another 5 minutes. Divide the dough into 4 equal parts. Roll the dough, one part at a time, into a rectangle about 12 x 10 inches. Keep the rest of the dough covered while working.

Drop 2 level teaspoons filling onto half of the rectangle, about 1 1/2 inches apart in 2 rows of 4 mounds each. Moisten the edges of the dough, and the dough between the rows of pumpkin mixture with water. Fold the other half of the dough up over the pumpkin mixture, pressing the dough down around the pumpkin. Cut between the rows of filling to make ravioli; press the edges together with a fork, or cut with a pastry wheel. Seal edges well. Repeat with the remaining dough and pumpkin filling. Place ravioli on towel. Let stand, turning once, until dry, about 30 minutes.

Cook ravioli in 4 quarts of boiling salted water until tender; drain carefully.

Nutrition:

Calories: 212 calories

Total Fat: 4.5 g

Cholesterol: 62 mg

Sodium: 574 mg

Total Carbohydrate: 35.7 g

Protein: 7.1 g

247.   Pumpkin Ravioli With Hazelnut Cream Sauce

Serving: 6

Ingredients

2 1/2 cups pumpkin puree

2 large carrots, cooked and pureed

2 onions, diced

1 clove garlic, minced

2 teaspoons ground coriander seed

1/2 teaspoon ground mace

1/2 teaspoon ground allspice

1 pinch ground cardamom

1 cup unsalted butter

1/3 pound grated Parmesan cheese

2 tablespoons real maple syrup

1 egg, beaten

2 1/2 pounds fresh pasta sheets

salt to taste

ground black pepper to taste

1 cup hazelnuts

3 cups heavy whipping cream

3 cloves garlic, minced

1 pinch cayenne pepper

1 pinch white pepper

salt to taste

2 cups shredded sorrel, stems removed

Direction

Sauté the onions, garlic, and spices in butter or margarine until the onions are soft. Stir together with the pureed vegetables. Add cheese, maple syrup, egg, salt, and black pepper. Adjust seasoning. Set the filling aside.

Preheat the oven to 400 degrees F (205 degrees C). Toast the hazelnuts in a shallow pan on the middle rack for 10 to 12 minutes, or until brown and fragrant. When they are cool enough to handle, wrap the nuts tightly in a lint-free towel, and vigorously rub nuts against the towel. Continue rubbing until the nuts are almost blond.

Cook the cream, garlic, cayenne, and white pepper over high heat; stir often, and adjust heat to keep the cream from boiling over. When the cream is thick enough to coat the back of a spoon, add a pinch salt. Adjust seasoning. Remove sauce from heat until you're ready to use it.

Lay one sheet of Fresh Pasta out on a flat surface. Spray with water to prevent drying, and to make it more flexible. Place half tablespoons of filling along the bottom edge of the pasta about 1/2 inch apart. For larger ravioli, use 1 tablespoon of filling, and leave 1 inch between dollops. Fold the pasta sheet over the filling, and cut apart with a ravioli cutter. Set the finished ravioli aside, and cover with a damp cloth. Repeat until filling and/or pasta is completely used.

Cook the ravioli in salted boiling water until al dente. Drain.

Meanwhile, reheat the sauce. Add the shredded sorrel to the sauce; cook just until it wilts -- about 30 seconds. Add half the hazelnuts, turn the heat off, and add the cooked ravioli. Stir gently, and serve immediately. Garnish with remaining hazelnuts.

248. Quick And Easy Greek Spaghetti

Serving: 4
Preparation Time: 15 Minutes
Cooking Time: 40 Minutes

Ingredients
1 (8 ounce) package spaghetti
extra-virgin olive oil, or as needed
1 (10 ounce) bag fresh spinach
1 (8 ounce) package sliced fresh mushrooms
1/4 cup red wine vinegar
1/4 cup balsamic vinegar
2 (14.5 ounce) cans diced tomatoes
1/4 cup chopped fresh basil
1 tablespoon chopped fresh parsley
1 (6 ounce) can sliced black olives, drained (optional)
2 ounces crumbled feta cheese, or to taste
Direction
Bring a large pot of lightly salted water to a rolling boil. Cook the spaghetti at a boil, stirring occasionally, until the tender yet firm to the bite, about 12 minutes; drain and set aside.

Heat olive oil in a large saucepan over medium heat; cook and stir the spinach and mushrooms in the hot oil until they give off their liquid, about 10 minutes. Add the red wine vinegar and balsamic vinegar; bring to a boil. Stir the tomatoes, basil, parsley, and black olives into the boiling mixture; continue cooking and stirring, until the flavors blend, about 10 more minutes.

Mix the cooked spaghetti into the tomato mixture and reduce heat to medium-low. Simmer the pasta and sauce until the flavors have blended, 8 to 10 minutes; stir the feta cheese into the pasta. Sprinkle with more feta cheese to serve.

Nutrition:
Calories: 413 calories
Total Fat: 11.7 g
Cholesterol: 13 mg
Sodium: 1095 mg
Total Carbohydrate: 60.7 g
Protein: 16.1 g

249.   Quick Gnocchi

Serving: 2
Preparation Time: 10 Minutes
Cooking Time: 5 Minutes

Ingredients

1 cup dry potato flakes

1 cup boiling water

1 egg, beaten

1 teaspoon salt

1/8 teaspoon ground black pepper

1 1/2 cups all-purpose flour

Direction

Place potato flakes in a medium-size bowl. Pour in boiling water; stir until blended. Let cool.

Stir in egg, salt, and pepper. Blend in enough flour to make a fairly stiff dough. Turn dough out on a well floured board. Knead lightly.

Divide dough in half. Shape each half into a long thin roll, the thickness of a breadstick. With a knife dipped in flour, cut into bite-size pieces.

Place a few gnocchi in boiling water. As the gnocchi rise to the top of the pot, remove them with a slotted spoon. Repeat until all are cooked.

Nutrition:

Calories: 462 calories

Total Fat: 3.5 g

Cholesterol: 93 mg

Sodium: 1225 mg

Total Carbohydrate: 91.3 g

Protein: 14.8 g

250. Quick Pasta Primavera

Serving: 5

Ingredients

5 ounces dry fettuccine pasta

1/4 cup water

2 cups fresh sliced mushrooms

9 ounces frozen French-style green beans

1/2 cup chopped red bell pepper

1 clove garlic, minced

1/4 teaspoon ground black pepper

1 (12 fluid ounce) can evaporated milk

4 teaspoons cornstarch

1/2 cup shredded mozzarella cheese

1 large tomato, cut into wedges

Direction

Bring a large pot of lightly salted water to a boil. Add pasta and cook for 8 to 10 minutes or until al dente; drain and reserve.

Meanwhile, in a medium sauce pan combine water, mushrooms, beans, red or green bell pepper, garlic, and ground black pepper. Bring to a boil; reduce heat. Cover and simmer for 4 minutes or until vegetables are tender; do not drain.

In a small bowl, combine milk and cornstarch; stir into vegetable mixture. Stir and cook over medium heat until thickened and bubbly. Cook and stir for 1 minute more; add cheese and stir until melted. Pour sauce over pasta and garnish with tomato wedges. Serve.

Nutrition:

Calories: 278 calories

Total Fat: 9.1 g

Cholesterol: 31 mg

Sodium: 156 mg

Total Carbohydrate: 36.9 g

Protein: 13.4 g

251.   Quick Stuffed Tomatoes

Serving: 4
Preparation Time: 25 Minutes
Cooking Time: 30 Minutes

Ingredients

4 large tomatoes

1 1/2 cups vegetable broth

1/2 cup sun-dried tomatoes, chopped

1 cup couscous

1/4 cup shredded nonfat mozzarella cheese

1/4 cup chopped fresh basil

2 tablespoons minced fresh mint leaves

1/4 teaspoon ground black pepper

Direction

Preheat oven to 375 degrees F (190 degree C).

Cut the fresh tomatoes crosswise in half and scoop out the pulp; set aside. Invert the tomato shells on paper towels to drain.

In a small saucepan, bring the broth and sun-dried tomatoes to a boil. Remove the saucepan from heat and stir in the couscous. Cover and let stand for 5 minutes.

Stir in the cheese, basil, mint and pepper. Then gently stir in the tomato pulp.

Place the tomato shells in an 11x7 inch baking dish. Spoon the couscous mixture into the shells, pressing the mixture firmly into the shells. Bake at 375 degrees F (190 degrees C) for 25 to 30 minutes or until heated through.

Nutrition:

Calories: 245 calories

Total Fat: 1.1 g

Cholesterol: 1 mg

Sodium: 284 mg

Total Carbohydrate: 47.7 g

Protein: 11.4 g

252. Quick Vegetarian Pasta With Spinach And Boursin

Serving: 1
Preparation Time: 5 Minutes
Cooking Time: 10 Minutes

Ingredients

1/3 (5.2 ounce) package garlic and herb cheese spread (such as Boursin®)

7 ounces frozen creamed spinach, thawed

5 1/2 ounces elbow macaroni

1 pinch freshly ground black pepper to taste

2 tablespoons cashews

Direction

Bring a large pot of lightly salted water to a boil. Cook elbow macaroni in the boiling water, stirring occasionally, until tender yet firm to the bite, about 8 minutes. Drain.

In the meantime, heat creamed spinach in a saucepan over medium-low heat until warm, about 5 minutes.

Mix drained macaroni with spinach and Boursin(R) cheese. Season with pepper and sprinkle with cashews.

Nutrition:

Calories: 1032 calories

Total Fat: 43.2 g

Cholesterol: 114 mg

Sodium: 1428 mg

Total Carbohydrate: 134.1 g

Protein: 30.9 g

253.   Reheating Pasta

Serving: 4
Preparation Time: 5 Minutes
Cooking Time: 10 Minutes

Ingredients

8 ounces dry pasta

3 tablespoons olive oil

Direction

Bring a large pot of lightly salted water to a boil. Add pasta and cook for 5 to 7 minutes or until still slightly less than al dente; drain. Rinse with cold water. Toss with olive oil. Cover and refrigerate until ready to use. To reheat, bring a large pot of water to a boil, add pasta and cook until hot, 1 to 2 minutes.

Nutrition:

Calories: 302 calories

Total Fat: 12.6 g

Cholesterol: 67 mg

Sodium: 15 mg

Total Carbohydrate: 39.2 g

Protein: 8.1 g

254. Restaurant Style Mac And Cheese

Serving: 4
Preparation Time: 15 Minutes
Cooking Time: 10 Minutes

Ingredients

1 1/2 cups macaroni

6 ounces processed cheese, shredded

1/2 cup shredded Cheddar cheese

2 tablespoons heavy cream

salt to taste

Direction

Bring a large pot of lightly salted water to a boil. Add pasta and cook for 8 to 10 minutes or until al dente; drain.

Return drained pasta to the pot. Mix in processed cheese, Cheddar cheese, and cream. Stir until cheeses melt. Sprinkle with salt.

Nutrition:

Calories: 376 calories

Total Fat: 18.9 g

Cholesterol: 59 mg

Sodium: 623 mg

Total Carbohydrate: 34 g

Protein: 17.1 g

255.   Rice Noodles With Shiitakes Choy And Chiles

Serving: 4

Ingredients

2 1/2 tablespoons soy sauce

3 tablespoons sake

2 tablespoons balsamic vinegar

2 teaspoons white sugar

3 tablespoons water

2 teaspoons cornstarch

1 tablespoon canola oil

2 tablespoons dark sesame oil

2 cloves garlic, sliced

6 whole dried red chile peppers, seeded and diced

1 tablespoon minced fresh ginger root

1 medium head bok choy, cut into 1 1/2 inch strips

20 fresh shiitake mushrooms, stemmed and quartered

8 green onions, halved lengthwise

2 (9 ounce) packages fresh rice noodles

2 tablespoons sesame seeds, toasted

Direction

In a small bowl, whisk together the soy sauce, sake or sherry, vinegar, sugar, water and cornstarch. In a large skillet or wok heat the oils over high heat. When the oil is nearly smoking, add the garlic and hot peppers. Take the skillet or wok off the heat after 10 seconds.

Reduce the heat to medium-high and return the skillet or wok to the heat. Add the ginger, bok choy, shiitakes, and green onions; cook for 3 minutes over high heat, stirring constantly. Add the fresh or soaked rice noodles and the soy sauce mixture; cook 2 minutes more or until the noodles are hot and tender. Serve the noodles immediately, topped with the toasted sesame seeds.

Nutrition:

Calories: 486 calories

Total Fat: 13.3 g

Cholesterol: 0 mg

Sodium: 728 mg

Total Carbohydrate: 77.5 g

Protein: 10.5 g

256. Rich Pasta For The Poor Kitchen

Serving: 4
Preparation Time: 10 Minutes
Cooking Time: 20 Minutes

Ingredients

1 (6 ounce) package dry spaghetti

8 tablespoons butter

2 tablespoons minced garlic

salt and freshly ground black pepper to taste

1 tablespoon chopped fresh parsley

cayenne pepper (optional)

1 cup grated Parmesan cheese

Direction

Bring a large pot of lightly salted water to a boil. Cook pasta for 8 to 10 minutes, or until al dente; drain.

Heat a skillet over medium-low heat. Melt butter with garlic very slowly to avoid burning the garlic. Season with salt, freshly ground black pepper, and parsley. Sprinkle with cayenne pepper to taste, if desired.

Toss pasta into the skillet until well-coated with butter. Increase heat to medium, and cook until pasta is heated through and has absorbed some of the butter. Adjust seasoning with salt and pepper, if necessary. Serve with grated Parmesan cheese.

Nutrition:

Calories: 453 calories

Total Fat: 29.5 g

Cholesterol: 79 mg

Sodium: 1055 mg

Total Carbohydrate: 33.8 g

Protein: 13.7 g

257. Roasted Butternut Squash And Garlic Lasagna

Serving: 12
Preparation Time: 30 Minutes
Cooking Time: 1 h 40 Minutes

Ingredients

3 pounds butternut squash, halved and seeded

3 tablespoons vegetable oil

1/2 teaspoon salt

1/4 cup unsalted butter

2 tablespoons minced garlic

1/4 cup all-purpose flour

1 quart milk

salt and ground black pepper to taste

1 cup heavy cream

9 no-cook lasagna noodles

1 1/3 cups finely grated Parmesan cheese

Direction

Preheat an oven to 450 degrees F (230 degrees C). Grease a baking sheet.

Brush the butternut squash halves with vegetable oil and season with salt. Roast in the preheated oven until golden and easily pierced with a knife, 45 to 50 minutes. Allow to cool for 15 to 20 minutes, then scoop the flesh into a bowl. Set aside.

Heat the butter in a large skillet over medium-low heat. Cook and stir garlic in the butter until softened. Stir in flour and cook for 3 minutes. Whisk in the milk until smooth. Bring to a simmer, and cook until thick, about 10 minutes, whisking occasionally. Stir in the butternut squash and season with salt and pepper. Sauce can be made 3 days ahead and refrigerated.

Reduce oven temperature to 375 degrees F (190 degrees C). Grease a 9x13 inch baking dish.

Beat the heavy cream until foamy in a large glass or metal mixing bowl. Gradually add the salt, continuing to beat until medium peaks form. Lift your beater or whisk straight up: the tip of the peak formed by the cream should curl over slightly. Set aside.

Pour 1 cup of the butternut sauce into the baking dish and place 3 lasagna noodles on top in a single layer. Spread half of the remaining sauce over the noodles and sprinkle with 1/2 cup of Parmesan cheese. Place another layer of noodles and spread the remaining sauce on top and sprinkle with 1/2 cup of Parmesan cheese. Place the final layer of noodles on top. Spread the whipped cream over the final layer of noodles making sure the pasta is completely covered. Sprinkle with the remaining 1/3 cup of Parmesan. Cover baking dish tightly with aluminum foil.

Bake in the preheated oven for 30 minutes. Remove foil and continue baking until the top is bubbly and golden brown, about 10 minutes. Allow to rest for 5 minutes before serving.

Nutrition:

Calories: 339 calories

Total Fat: 19.3 g

Cholesterol: 52 mg

Sodium: 280 mg

Total Carbohydrate: 33.5 g

Protein: 10.4 g

258.   Roasted Butternut Squash And Spinach Lasagna

Serving: 10
Preparation Time: 30 Minutes
Cooking Time: 1 h 59 Minutes

Ingredients

1 butternut squash - peeled, seeded, and cubed

1 tablespoon olive oil, or to taste

1 tablespoon chopped garlic

3 dashes ground sage

1 pinch seasoned salt (such as The Chef's Miracle Blend®), or to taste

Sauce:

1/4 cup butter

2 teaspoons chopped garlic

1/4 cup all-purpose flour

3 cups milk

1 pinch salt and ground black pepper to taste

1 teaspoon chili powder

3 dashes ground sage

1/2 teaspoon dried rosemary

Cheese Mixture:

1 (16 ounce) container ricotta cheese

2 cups shredded mozzarella cheese, divided

1 (10 ounce) package frozen chopped spinach, drained and squeezed dry

1 egg

1/4 cup grated Parmesan cheese

9 no-boil lasagna noodles

Direction

Preheat oven to 400 degrees F (200 degrees C).

Toss butternut squash with olive oil, 1 tablespoon garlic, ground sage, and seasoned salt in a 9x11-inch baking dish until coated.

Roast in the preheated oven, stirring every 20 minutes, until butternut squash is tender, about 1 hour.

Reduce oven temperature to 375 degrees F (190 degrees C).

Melt butter in a large saucepan over medium heat. Add garlic; cook and stir until fragrant, about 1 minute. Whisk in flour until a smooth paste forms. Slowly pour in milk; season with salt and pepper. Cook and stir sauce until thick and bubbling, 8 to 10 minutes.

Remove sauce from heat; stir in roasted butternut squash, chili powder, ground sage, and rosemary. Puree sauce with an immersion blender until smooth.

Mix ricotta cheese, 1 1/2 cup mozzarella cheese, spinach, egg, and Parmesan cheese together in a bowl.

Spread 1/2 cup sauce in the bottom of the baking dish. Lay 3 lasagna noodles on top. Spread 1/3 of the ricotta cheese mixture over the noodles. Repeat layers twice more, ending with remaining sauce. Sprinkle remaining 1/2 cup mozzarella cheese on top. Cover baking dish with aluminum foil.

Bake in the preheated oven until mozzarella cheese is melted, about 40 minutes. Uncover and continue baking until bubbly, about 10 minutes more.

Nutrition:

Calories: 345 calories

Total Fat: 16.6 g

Cholesterol: 68 mg

Sodium: 367 mg

Total Carbohydrate: 33 g

Protein: 18.7 g

259.   Roasted Eggplant Lasagna

Serving: 6
Preparation Time: 25 Minutes
Cooking Time: 1 hours

Ingredients

1 large eggplant, peeled and cut into 1/4-inch slices

salt to taste

2 tablespoons olive oil, or as needed

1 (16 ounce) container ricotta cheese

2 cups shredded Italian cheese blend

1 egg

2 cloves garlic, minced

2 sprigs fresh oregano, chopped

3 sprigs fresh thyme, chopped

10 grinds fresh black pepper

2 1/2 cups tomato sauce

1 (10 ounce) package frozen chopped spinach, thawed and drained

6 slices part-skim mozzarella cheese

Direction

Preheat oven to 450 degrees F (230 degrees C).

Place eggplant slices on a wire rack; sprinkle with salt. Let sit until some liquid starts beading on slices, about 20 minutes. Rinse salt off eggplant slices and pat dry. Brush olive oil over both sides of each slice. Arrange eggplant slices on a baking sheet.

Roast in the preheated oven for 10 to 15 minutes. Flip eggplant slices and continue roasting until slices are tender and lightly browned, 15 to 20 more minutes. Remove eggplant from oven and reduce temperature to 350 degrees F (175 degrees C).

Mix ricotta cheese, Italian cheese blend, egg, garlic, oregano, thyme, and black pepper together in a bowl.

Line a 9-inch square pan with aluminum foil. Coat the bottom of the pan with about 1/2 cup tomato sauce; top with 1/2 of the eggplant slices. Layer eggplant slices with 1/2 of the spinach, 1/2 of the ricotta mixture, and 1/2 of the remaining tomato sauce. Continue layering with remaining ingredients, ending with sauce. Top with mozzarella slices. Cover pan with aluminum foil.

Bake in the preheated oven for 30 minutes. Remove aluminum foil and continue baking until cheese is brown and bubbling, 5 to 10 more minutes.

Nutrition:

Calories: 432 calories

Total Fat: 26.9 g

Cholesterol: 102 mg

Sodium: 1179 mg

Total Carbohydrate: 21.7 g

Protein: 29.8 g

260.   Roasted Veggie Pasta

Serving: 3
Preparation Time: 15 Minutes
Cooking Time: 15 Minutes

Ingredients

1/4 pound fresh asparagus

2 red bell pepper, sliced

1/4 pound crimini mushrooms, sliced

10 cloves roasted garlic, chopped

1/2 tomato, quartered

1/2 teaspoon chopped fresh rosemary

1/2 teaspoon chopped fresh oregano

2 tablespoons olive oil

8 ounces dry fettuccini noodles

1/4 cup grated Parmesan cheese

2 tablespoons tapenade

Direction

Preheat oven to 350 degrees F (175 degrees C). Prepare asparagus by trimming woody base and cutting diagonally into 4 inch pieces.

In a roasting pan, combine asparagus, bell pepper, mushrooms, roasted garlic and tomato. Sprinkle with rosemary and oregano, then drizzle with olive oil. Bake in preheated oven for 15 minutes.

Bring a large pot of lightly salted water to a boil. Add pasta and cook for 8 to 10 minutes or until al dente; drain. Toss with Parmesan cheese, tapenade and roasted vegetables.

Nutrition:

Calories: 456 calories

Total Fat: 14.6 g

Cholesterol: 6 mg

Sodium: 213 mg

Total Carbohydrate: 66.7 g

Protein: 16.8 g

261.   Rustica

Serving: 1
Preparation Time: 10 Minutes
Cooking Time: 8 Minutes

Ingredients

3/4 cup rotini pasta

1 clove garlic, minced

2 teaspoons olive oil

2 tablespoons chopped fresh parsley

salt and ground black pepper to taste

1/4 cup grated Parmesan cheese

Direction

Bring a large pot of lightly salted water to a boil; add the rotini and cook until al dente, 8 to 10 minutes; drain.

Heat the oil in a skillet over medium heat. Cook the garlic in the hot oil until it begins to brown, 3 to 5 minutes; stir in the parsley and cook another 30 seconds; remove from heat immediately and spoon over the drained pasta; season with salt and pepper. Top with Parmesan cheese.

Nutrition:

Calories: 433 calories

Total Fat: 17.7 g

Cholesterol: 22 mg

Sodium: 391 mg

Total Carbohydrate: 49.5 g

Protein: 18.2 g

262.   Salsa Di Noci

Serving: 4
Preparation Time: 10 Minutes
Cooking Time: 15 Minutes

Ingredients

3 cups water, or as needed

1 1/2 cups walnuts

2 cloves garlic, peeled

1 pinch sea salt

1 teaspoon chopped fresh marjoram

1 teaspoon chopped fresh thyme

1 teaspoon chopped fresh oregano

1/2 cup extra-virgin olive oil

3/4 cup heavy cream

1 cup finely grated Pecorino Romano cheese

freshly ground black pepper to taste

sea salt to taste

1 (16 ounce) box dry fettuccine pasta

1/2 bunch fresh chives, finely chopped

Direction

Bring water to a boil in a small saucepan. Add walnuts and cook until they have softened slightly, about 5 minutes. Drain and set aside.

Combine garlic and 1 pinch sea salt in the bowl of a mortar and pestle. Grind to create a thick paste. Add walnuts, marjoram, thyme, and oregano. Grind until combined and slightly creamy, but still coarse.

Transfer the walnut mixture to a large bowl. Slowly whisk in olive oil to form a thick emulsion. Add heavy cream and Pecorino Romano cheese, whisk until combined. Season with black pepper and sea salt to taste.

Fill a large pot with lightly salted water and bring to a rolling boil. Stir in the fettuccine, return to a boil, and cook pasta over medium heat until cooked through but still firm to the bite, about 8 minutes. Drain.

Toss walnut sauce with pasta. Garnish with fresh chives.

Nutrition:

Calories: 1116 calories

Total Fat: 74.7 g

Cholesterol: 71 mg

Sodium: 370 mg

Total Carbohydrate: 90.4 g

Protein: 26.3 g

263.   Sauceless Garden Lasagna

Serving: 6
Preparation Time: 20 Minutes
Cooking Time: 45 Minutes

Ingredients

1 medium zucchini, halved lengthwise and sliced

1/3 cup chopped red onion

1 cup shredded mozzarella cheese, divided

1/2 cup crumbled feta cheese

2 portobello mushrooms, sliced

4 cups fresh baby spinach

1/4 cup chopped fresh basil

1 tablespoon chopped fresh oregano

3 cloves garlic, minced

3 tablespoons olive oil

1/4 cup balsamic vinegar

1 teaspoon sugar

1/2 teaspoon salt

1/4 teaspoon freshly ground black pepper

1 (8 ounce) package no-boil lasagna noodles

9 roma (plum) tomatoes, thinly sliced

Direction

Preheat the oven to 350 degrees F (175 degrees C). Lightly coat a 9x9 inch baking dish with cooking spray.

In a large bowl, toss together the zucchini, mushrooms, spinach, garlic, red onion, 1/2 cup mozzarella cheese, and feta cheese. Drizzle with olive oil and balsamic vinegar, and stir in basil, oregano, sugar, salt and pepper. Stir the mixture until evenly blended.

Place a layer of lasagna noodles into the bottom of the prepared pan. Make a layer of tomato slices over the noodles. Spread a generous amount of the spinach mixture over the tomatoes. Don't worry, it shrinks a lot while cooking. Lay slices of tomatoes over the spinach mixture, then another layer of noodles. Start with another layer of tomatoes on top of the noodles, and repeat layering until the dish is heaped with lasagna, ending with the vegetable mixture. Sprinkle remaining cheese on the top.

Bake for 35 to 45 minutes in the preheated oven, until noodles, and vegetables are tender. Let stand for a few minutes to set, then slice and serve.

Nutrition:

Calories: 286 calories

Total Fat: 15.5 g

Cholesterol: 32 mg

Sodium: 576 mg

Total Carbohydrate: 25.3 g

Protein: 12.9 g

264.   Sauerkraut Filling For Pierogi

Serving: 6

Ingredients

2 tablespoons vegetable oil

1 cup chopped onion

1 cup chopped mushrooms

14 ounces sauerkraut - drained, rinsed and minced

1/4 teaspoon salt

1/4 teaspoon ground black pepper

2 tablespoons sour cream

Direction

In a large skillet, heat oil over a medium flame. Add onions and mushrooms, and cook until tender but not brown. Stir in sauerkraut, 1/4 teaspoon salt, and 1/4 teaspoon black pepper. Cook for 6 to 10 minutes. Remove from heat, and stir in 2 tablespoons sour cream.

Nutrition:

Calories: 77 calories

Total Fat: 5.7 g

Cholesterol: 2 mg

Sodium: 533 mg

Total Carbohydrate: 5.9 g

Protein: 1.4 g

265.   Slow Cooker Spinach And Crab Lasagna

Serving: 8
Preparation Time: 15 Minutes
Cooking Time: 2 h 45 Minutes

Ingredients

1 (16 ounce) jar Alfredo sauce

1 (16 ounce) package dried lasagna noodles

1 bunch fresh spinach, chopped

15 fresh mushrooms, sliced

1 (8 ounce) package imitation crabmeat

1 (12 ounce) container cottage cheese

12 ounces ricotta cheese

1 1/2 cups shredded mozzarella cheese

Direction

Pour half the jar of Alfredo sauce into the slow cooker; top with a layer of lasagna noodles. Spread a layer of spinach, a layer of mushrooms, and a layer of crabmeat, respectively, over lasagna noodle layer. Spoon half the cottage cheese and half the ricotta cheese over crabmeat layer. Repeat layering with remaining ingredients, ending with a final layer of noodles and Alfredo sauce.

Cook on High for 2 hours 15 minutes. Sprinkle mozzarella cheese over lasagna on cook on High until cheese is melted, about 30 minutes more.

Nutrition:

Calories: 566 calories

Total Fat: 26.9 g

Cholesterol: 62 mg

Sodium: 1180 mg

Total Carbohydrate: 54.3 g

Protein: 29.9 g

266. Smothered Mexican Lasagna

Serving: 6
Preparation Time: 20 Minutes
Cooking Time: 25 Minutes

Ingredients

1 1/2 pounds ground turkey

1 bunch green onions, chopped

1 (1.25 ounce) package taco seasoning mix

2 cups water

1 (14.5 ounce) can diced tomatoes, undrained

1 (4 ounce) can diced green chile peppers, undrained

1 (15 ounce) container ricotta cheese

2 eggs

8 (10 inch) flour tortillas

1 (8 ounce) container sour cream

1/4 cup salsa

Direction

Preheat oven to 400 degrees F (200 degrees C). Place ground turkey in a large, deep skillet. Cook over medium high heat until evenly brown. Stir in green onions, taco seasoning mix, water, diced tomatoes with juice, and green chiles with juice. Reduce heat to medium.

In a medium bowl, mix together ricotta and eggs. Place 2 tortillas in the bottom of a 9x13 inch pan. Spread 1/4 of the ricotta mixture on tortillas. Spoon 1/4 of the meat mixture over the cheese. Repeat layers until all is used up.

Bake in preheated oven for 20 minutes, or until sauce is bubbly. In a small bowl, mix together sour cream and salsa. Serve in a bowl on the side.

Nutrition:

Calories: 716 calories

Total Fat: 31.9 g

Cholesterol: 190 mg

Sodium: 1660 mg

Total Carbohydrate: 63.9 g

Protein: 40.5 g

267.   Special Mushroom Lasagna

Serving: 12
Preparation Time: 02 h 00 Minutes
Cooking Time: 55 Minutes

Ingredients

6 tablespoons butter, divided

3-1/2 pounds sliced baby portobello mushrooms

1 large onion, thinly sliced

1 cup marsala wine

8 garlic cloves, minced, divided

2 tablespoons dried minced onion

12 uncooked lasagna noodles

5 tablespoons all-purpose flour

1 teaspoon onion powder

1/2 teaspoon white pepper

1/2 teaspoon ground nutmeg

1/4 teaspoon cayenne pepper

3 cups whole milk

1 package (8 ounces) cream cheese, softened

1/2 cup minced chives

1 jar (2 ounces) diced pimientos, drained

1 tablespoon lemon juice

1/2 teaspoon grated lemon zest

1/2 teaspoon salt

2 cups grated Parmesan cheese

6 ounces fresh crabmeat, optional

CRUMB TOPPING:

1 French bread demi-baguette (about 4 ounces)

1/2 cup grated Parmesan cheese

2 tablespoons butter, melted

1/2 cup minced chives

Direction

In a Dutch oven, melt 2 tablespoons butter over medium heat. Add mushrooms and onion; sauté until tender. Add wine, four minced garlic cloves and minced onion; bring to a boil. Cook until liquid is absorbed, about 30 minutes. Meanwhile, cook lasagna noodles according to package directions. In a large saucepan over medium heat, melt remaining butter. Stir in next five ingredients and remaining garlic until blended; gradually add milk. Bring to a boil; cook and stir until thickened, 1-2 minutes. Stir in next six ingredients until blended. Remove from heat. Preheat oven to 350 degrees. Drain lasagna noodles. Spread 1 cup cream cheese sauce in a greased 13x9-in. baking pan. Layer with three noodles, 1 cup sauce, a third of the mushroom mixture and 2/3 cup Parmesan cheese. Repeat layers, adding crabmeat, if desired, between mushrooms and Parmesan. Layer with three more noodles, 1 cup sauce, remaining mushroom mixture and remaining Parmesan cheese. Top with remaining noodles and sauce. For crumb topping, pulse baguette, cheese and butter in a food processor until finely chopped. Stir in chives. Sprinkle over lasagna. Bake, covered, about 50 minutes. Uncover; bake until bubbly, 5-10 minutes longer. Let stand 10 minutes before cutting.

Nutrition:

Calories: 423 calories

Total Fat: 22g

Cholesterol: 60mg

Sodium: 616mg

Total Carbohydrate: 41g

Protein: 17g

Fiber: 3g

268.   Spinach Alfredo Lasagna

Serving: 8-10
Preparation Time: 20 Minutes
Cooking Time: 45 Minutes

Ingredients

12 ounces uncooked lasagna noodles

1 pound Jones No Sugar Pork Sausage Roll sausage

1 package (10 ounces) frozen chopped spinach, thawed and squeezed dry

1 jar (15 ounces) Alfredo sauce

1/2 teaspoon salt

1/4 teaspoon pepper

1 large egg

2 cups shredded cheddar cheese

1 carton (15 ounces) ricotta cheese

1/2 cup grated Parmesan cheese

1 cup shredded mozzarella cheese

Direction

Soak the noodles in hot water for 15 minutes. Meanwhile, in a large skillet, cook the sausage over medium heat until no longer pink. Drain noodles; set aside. Drain sausage; add the spinach, Alfredo sauce, salt and pepper. In a small bowl, combine the egg and cheddar, ricotta and Parmesan cheeses. In an ungreased 13x9-in. baking dish, layer a third of the sausage mixture, noodles and cheese mixture. Repeat layers twice. Sprinkle with mozzarella cheese. Cover and bake at 350 degrees for 45 minutes. Let stand for 15 minutes before cutting.

Nutrition:

Calories: 490 calories

Total Fat: 29g

Cholesterol: 104mg

Sodium: 828mg

Total Carbohydrate: 34g

Protein: 25g

Fiber: 2g

269. Spinach And Turkey Sausage Lasagna

Serving: 12
Preparation Time: 60 Minutes
Cooking Time: 55 Minutes
Ingredients

3 tablespoons butter

1/3 cup all-purpose flour

1/2 teaspoon salt

1/4 teaspoon pepper

3 cups fat-free milk

3 ounces reduced-fat cream cheese, cubed

3/4 cup grated Parmesan cheese

1 pound Italian turkey sausage links, casings removed and crumbled

1 medium onion, chopped

4 garlic cloves, minced

1 teaspoon dried oregano

1 teaspoon dried marjoram

1/2 teaspoon fennel seed, crushed

1 jar (7 ounces) roasted sweet red peppers, drained and chopped

1/2 cup white wine or reduced-sodium chicken broth

2 packages (10 ounces each) frozen chopped spinach, thawed and squeezed dry

3/4 cup 2% cottage cheese

1/4 teaspoon ground nutmeg

9 lasagna noodles, cooked, rinsed and drained

1/2 cup shredded part-skim mozzarella cheese

Direction

In a large saucepan, melt butter. Stir in flour, salt and pepper until smooth; gradually stir in milk. Bring to a boil; cook and stir for 1-2 minutes or until thickened. Stir in cream cheese until melted. Stir in Parmesan cheese just until melted. Remove from the heat; set aside. In a large nonstick skillet coated with cooking spray, cook sausage and onion over medium heat until sausage is no longer pink. Add the garlic, oregano, marjoram and fennel; cook 1 minute longer. Add roasted peppers and wine. Bring to a boil. Reduce heat; simmer, uncovered, for 3-5 minutes or until liquid is reduced to 3 tablespoons. Remove from the heat; set aside. In a small bowl, combine the spinach, cottage cheese and nutmeg. Spread 1/2 cup cheese sauce in a 13-in. x 9-in. baking dish coated with cooking spray. Top with three noodles, half of the sausage mixture, half of the spinach mixture and 1 cup sauce; repeat layers. Top with remaining noodles and sauce. Sprinkle with mozzarella cheese. Cover and bake at 375 degrees for 40 minutes. Uncover; bake 15-20 minutes longer or until heated through and top is lightly browned. Let stand for 10 minutes before cutting.

Nutrition:

Calories: 279 calories

Total Fat: 11g

Cholesterol: 43mg

Sodium: 664mg

Total Carbohydrate: 27g

Protein: 19g

Fiber: 3g

270.   Spinach Lasagna

Serving: 8

Ingredients

1 (1.5 ounce) package spaghetti sauce mix

1 (6 ounce) can tomato paste

1 (8 ounce) can tomato sauce

1 3/4 cups water

2 eggs

1 pint ricotta cheese

1/2 teaspoon salt

1 (10 ounce) package frozen chopped spinach, thawed and drained

1/2 cup Parmesan cheese

8 ounces sliced mozzarella cheese

8 lasagna noodles

Direction

Preheat oven to 350 degrees F (175 degrees C). Lightly grease one 13x9 inch baking dish.

In a medium saucepan, combine spaghetti sauce mix, tomato sauce, tomato paste and water. Bring to a boil over medium heat then remove from heat and let cool.

In a medium bowl, beat the eggs and combine them with the ricotta or cottage cheese, salt, spinach and 1/4 cup of the Parmesan cheese.

Spread one half cup tomato sauce mixture into the prepared baking dish. Place half the uncooked noodles over the sauce, spread with half the spinach mixture, half the mozzarella cheese, and half of the tomato sauce. Repeat layers, using remaining ingredients. Top with remaining Parmesan cheese.

Cover dish securely with aluminum foil and bake for in the preheated oven 1 hour. Let stand 10 minutes before cutting and serving.

Nutrition:

Calories: 346 calories

Total Fat: 13.8 g

Cholesterol: 91 mg

Sodium: 1159 mg

Total Carbohydrate: 32.7 g

Protein: 24.7 g

271.   Spinach Lasagna

Serving: 12
Preparation Time: 35 Minutes
Cooking Time: 1 hours

Ingredients

20 lasagna noodles

2 tablespoons olive oil

1 cup chopped fresh mushrooms

1 cup chopped onion

1 tablespoon minced garlic

2 cups fresh spinach

3 cups ricotta cheese

2/3 cup grated Romano cheese

1 teaspoon salt

1 teaspoon dried oregano

1 teaspoon dried basil leaves

1/2 teaspoon ground black pepper

1 egg

3 cups shredded mozzarella cheese

3 cups tomato pasta sauce

1 cup grated Parmesan cheese

Direction

Preheat oven to 350 degrees F (175 degrees C).

Bring a large pot of lightly salted water to a boil. Add lasagna noodles and cook for 8 to 10 minutes or until al dente; drain.

In a skillet over medium-high heat, cook mushrooms, onions, and garlic in olive oil until onions are tender. Drain excess liquid and cool. Boil spinach for 5 minutes. Drain, then squeeze out excess liquid. Chop spinach.

Combine ricotta cheese, Romano cheese, spinach, salt, oregano, basil, pepper, and egg in a bowl. Add cooled mushroom mixture. Beat with an electric mixer on low speed for 1 minute. Lay 5 lasagna noodles in bottom of a 9x13 inch baking dish. Spread one third of the cheese/spinach mixture over noodles. Sprinkle 1 cup mozzarella cheese and 1/3 cup Parmesan cheese on top. Spread 1 cup pasta sauce over cheese. Repeat layering 2 times.

Cover dish with aluminum foil and bake in a preheated oven for 1 hour. Cool 15 minutes before serving.

Nutrition:

Calories: 360 calories

Total Fat: 13.5 g

Cholesterol: 48 mg

Sodium: 875 mg

Total Carbohydrate: 41.2 g

Protein: 19 g

272.   Spinach Lasagna Rollups

Serving: 6
Preparation Time: 30 Minutes
Cooking Time: 25 Minutes

Ingredients

12 uncooked lasagna noodles

2 large eggs, lightly beaten

1 package (10 ounces) frozen chopped spinach, thawed and squeezed dry

2-1/2 cups whole-milk ricotta cheese

2-1/2 cups shredded part-skim mozzarella cheese

1/2 cup grated Parmesan cheese

1/4 teaspoon salt

1/4 teaspoon pepper

1/4 teaspoon ground nutmeg

1 jar (24 ounces) meatless pasta sauce

Direction

Preheat oven to 375 degrees. Cook and drain noodles according to package directions. Meanwhile, mix eggs, spinach, cheeses and seasonings. Pour 1 cup pasta sauce into an ungreased 13x9-in. baking dish. Spread 1/3 cup cheese mixture over each noodle; roll up and place over sauce, seam side down. Top with remaining sauce. Bake, covered, 20 minutes. Uncover; bake until heated through, 5-10 minutes.

Nutrition:

Calories: 569 calories

Total Fat: 22g

Cholesterol: 145mg

Sodium: 1165mg

Total Carbohydrate: 57g

Protein: 38g

Fiber: 5g

273.   Spinach Vegetable Lasagna

Serving: 12
Preparation Time: 30 Minutes
Cooking Time: 25 Minutes

Ingredients

3 tablespoons butter

1/2 cup all-purpose flour

2-3/4 cups fat-free milk, divided

1-1/2 cups plus 2 tablespoons grated Parmesan cheese, divided

3 tablespoons Dijon mustard

1/2 teaspoon salt, divided

1/4 teaspoon hot pepper sauce

1/2 pound sliced fresh mushrooms

2 medium onions, chopped

2 cups chopped carrots

4 garlic cloves, minced

1 tablespoon olive oil

1 pound fresh spinach, chopped

9 lasagna noodles, cooked, rinsed and drained

Direction

In a large saucepan, melt butter. Stir in flour until smooth. Add 2-1/2 cups milk. Bring to a boil; cook and stir for 1-2 minutes or until thickened. Remove from the heat. Stir in 1-1/2 cups Parmesan cheese, mustard, 1/4 teaspoon salt and hot pepper sauce; set aside. In a large nonstick skillet, sauté the mushrooms, onions, carrots and garlic in oil until tender. Stir in spinach and remaining salt. Cook and stir for 2 minutes or until spinach is wilted; drain. Remove from the heat; stir in 1-1/2 cups cheese sauce. Combine the remaining cheese sauce and milk. Spread half of the cheese sauce in a 13-in. x 9-in. baking dish coated with cooking spray. Top with three noodles and half the vegetable mixture; repeat. Top with remaining noodles and cheese sauce. Sprinkle with remaining cheese. Bake, uncovered, at 375 degrees for 25-30 minutes or until heated through. Let stand for 10 minutes before cutting.

Nutrition:

Calories: 222 calories

Total Fat: 8g

Cholesterol: 17mg

Sodium: 496mg

Total Carbohydrate: 27g

Protein: 12g

Fiber: 3g

274.   Spinach Venison Lasagna

Serving: 8
Preparation Time: 40 Minutes
Cooking Time: 45 Minutes

Ingredients

1/4 cup chopped onion

2 tablespoons butter

2 cans (8 ounces each) tomato sauce

1/2 cup water

1 tablespoon barbecue sauce

1 teaspoon each Worcestershire sauce and dried basil

1 bay leaf

1/4 teaspoon each garlic powder, ground cloves, ground allspice and dried oregano

WHITE SAUCE:

1 can (4 ounces) mushroom stems and pieces, drained

1/4 cup chopped onion

1/3 cup all-purpose flour

2 cups milk

12 lasagna noodles, cooked and drained

2 packages (10 ounces each) frozen chopped spinach, thawed and squeezed dry

1 cup 1% cottage cheese

3 cups shredded part-skim mozzarella cheese

2 pounds ground venison, cooked and drained

1 cup shredded cheddar cheese

Direction

In a large skillet, sauté onion in butter until tender. Stir in tomato sauce, water, barbecue sauce, Worcestershire sauce and seasonings. Bring to a boil. Reduce heat. Cover; simmer for 30 minutes. Meanwhile, in a saucepan, sauté mushrooms and onion in butter until tender. Stir in flour. Gradually whisk in milk until blended. Bring to a boil; cook and stir for 2 minutes or until thickened. Discard bay leaf. Spread 1/2 cup tomato sauce into a greased 13-in. x 9-in. baking dish; top with four noodles. Layer with 1 cup spinach, 1/2 cup cottage cheese, half of white sauce, 1 cup mozzarella cheese, half of venison and 1/2 cup cheddar cheese. Repeat layers once. Top with remaining noodles, tomato sauce and mozzarella cheese. Cover; bake at 350 degrees for 35 minutes. Uncover; bake 10-15 minutes longer. Let stand 10 minutes.

Nutrition:

Calories:

Total Fat: g

Cholesterol: mg

Sodium: mg

Total Carbohydrate: g

Protein: g

Fiber: g

275.   Summer Garden Lasagna

Serving: 6
Preparation Time: 45 Minutes
Cooking Time: 1 h 15 Minutes

Ingredients

1 teaspoon olive oil

1 (16 ounce) package lasagna noodles

3 ears corn, shucked

1 tablespoon extra-virgin olive oil, divided

2 zucchini, sliced into long ribbons using a vegetable peeler, discarding the seedy core

salt and ground black pepper to taste

1/4 cup chopped onion

1 clove garlic

1 (24 ounce) jar marinara sauce, divided

2 tablespoons heavy whipping cream

2 cups ricotta cheese

1 (9 ounce) package frozen chopped spinach, thawed and drained

1 cup shredded mozzarella cheese

1/4 cup grated Parmigiano-Reggiano cheese

Direction

Preheat oven to 375 degrees F (190 degrees C). Grease an 8x6-inch baking dish with 1 teaspoon olive oil.

Bring a large pot of lightly salted water to a boil. Cook lasagna in the boiling water, stirring occasionally until cooked through but firm to the bite, about 8 minutes. Drain.

Bring another large pot of lightly salted water to a boil. Cook corn in the boiling water until cooked through, about 5 minutes. Cut kernels from the cobs and discard cobs.

Heat 1 1/2 teaspoons extra virgin olive oil in a large skillet over medium-high heat. Sauté zucchini ribbons with a pinch of salt and black pepper in hot oil until golden and cooked through, about 5 minutes.

Heat remaining extra virgin olive oil in a large saucepan over medium heat. Cook and stir onion in hot oil until translucent, 5 to 7 minutes. Add garlic; cook and stir until fragrant, about 1 minute. Pour 1/3 of the marinara sauce into the onion mixture; bring to a simmer, reduce heat to low, stir in cream, and cook until sauce is slightly reduced, 5 to 10 minutes.

Pour 1/3 of the marinara sauce into the bottom of the prepared baking dish. Place a layer of lasagna noodles over the marinara sauce, trimming noodles as necessary to fit the baking dish. Spread zucchini ribbons over the noodle layer and top with another layer of lasagna noodles.

Spread ricotta cheese over the lasagna noodles and place another layer of noodles atop the cheese. Pour marinara-cream mixture over the noodles and top with corn kernels.

Place a layer of lasagna noodles over the corn kernels and top noodles with spinach. Add a final layer of noodles and top noodles with remaining marinara sauce. Sprinkle mozzarella cheese and Parmigiano-Reggiano cheese over the top. Cover the baking dish with aluminum foil.

Bake in the preheated oven for 30 minutes. Remove the aluminum foil and continue baking lasagna until cheese is browned and beginning to bubble, about 15 minutes more.

Nutrition:

Calories: 536 calories

Total Fat: 14.5 g

Cholesterol: 24 mg

Sodium: 678 mg

Total Carbohydrate: 83.9 g

Protein: 21.8 g

276. Swiss Cheese Lasagna

Serving: 12
Preparation Time: 60 Minutes
Cooking Time: 40 Minutes

Ingredients

1 pound ground beef

1 large onion, chopped

1 garlic clove, minced

3 cups water

1 can (12 ounces) tomato paste

2 teaspoons salt

1/2 to 1 teaspoon dried rosemary, crushed

1/4 teaspoon pepper

1 package (8 ounces) lasagna noodles

8 ounces sliced Swiss cheese

1-1/2 cups (12 ounces each) 4% cottage cheese

1/2 cup shredded part-skim mozzarella cheese

Direction

In a large skillet, cook the beef, onion and garlic over medium heat until meat is no longer pink; drain. Stir in the water, tomato paste, salt, rosemary and pepper. Bring to a boil. Reduce heat; simmer, uncovered, for 30 minutes. Meanwhile, cook lasagna noodles according to package directions; drain. In a greased 13-in. x 9-in. baking dish, layer a third of the meat sauce, noodles and Swiss cheese. Repeat layers. Top with cottage cheese and the remaining Swiss cheese, noodles and sauce. Sprinkle with mozzarella cheese. Cover and bake at 350 degrees for 30 minutes. Uncover; bake 10-15 minutes longer or until bubbly. Let stand for 10 minutes before serving.

Nutrition:

Calories: 275 calories

Total Fat: 11g

Cholesterol: 48mg

Sodium: 596mg

Total Carbohydrate: 23g

Protein: 20g

Fiber: 3g

277.   Three Cheese Rice Lasagna

Serving: 6
Preparation Time: 15 Minutes
Cooking Time: 10 Minutes

Ingredients

1 jar (14 ounces) meatless spaghetti sauce

1 jar (4-1/2 ounces) sliced mushrooms, drained

1 cup (8 ounces) 1% cottage cheese

1 cup shredded part-skim mozzarella cheese

1 large egg white

3 cups cooked long grain rice

2 tablespoons grated Parmesan cheese

Direction

In a small bowl, combine spaghetti sauce and mushrooms; set aside. In another bowl, combine the cottage cheese, mozzarella cheese and egg white. In a microwave-safe 8-in. square baking dish coated with cooking spray, layer a third of the sauce, half of the rice and half of the cottage cheese mixture; repeat layers. Top with the remaining sauce. Microwave at 50% power for 7-12 minutes or until heated through. Sprinkle with Parmesan cheese. Let stand for 5 minutes before serving.

Nutrition:

Calories: 238 calories

Total Fat: 6g

Cholesterol: 14mg

Sodium: 664mg

Total Carbohydrate: 31g

Protein: 15g

Fiber: 2g

278.   Tofu Spinach Lasagna

Serving: 12
Preparation Time: 45 Minutes
Cooking Time: 30 Minutes

Ingredients

9 lasagna noodles

1 medium onion, chopped

3 garlic cloves, minced

1 tablespoon olive oil

2 cups sliced fresh mushrooms

1 package (14 ounces) firm tofu

1 carton (15 ounces) part-skim ricotta cheese

1/2 cup minced fresh parsley

1 teaspoon salt, divided

2 packages (10 ounces each) frozen chopped spinach, thawed and squeezed dry

1-3/4 cups marinara or meatless spaghetti sauce

1 cup shredded part-skim mozzarella cheese

1/3 cup shredded Parmesan cheese

Direction

Cook noodles according to package directions. Meanwhile, in a large nonstick skillet, sauté onion and garlic in oil for 1 minute. Add mushrooms; sauté until tender. Set aside. Drain tofu, reserving 2 tablespoons liquid. Place tofu and reserved liquid in a food processor; cover and process until blended. Add ricotta cheese; cover and process for 1-2 minutes or until smooth. Transfer to a large bowl; stir in the parsley, 1/2 teaspoon salt and mushroom mixture. Combine spinach and remaining salt; set aside. Drain noodles. Spread half of the marinara sauce into a 13x9-in. baking dish coated with cooking spray. Layer with three noodles, half of the tofu mixture and half of the spinach mixture. Repeat layers of noodles, tofu and spinach. Top with remaining noodles and marinara sauce. Sprinkle with cheeses. Bake, uncovered, at 350 degrees for 30-35 minutes or until heated through and cheese is melted. Let stand for 10 minutes before cutting.

Nutrition:

Calories: 227 calories

Total Fat: 8g

Cholesterol: 18mg

Sodium: 429mg

Total Carbohydrate: 25g

Protein: 15g

Fiber: 3g

279.   Tomato French Bread Lasagna

Serving: 10
Preparation Time: 30 Minutes
Cooking Time: 40 Minutes

Ingredients

1 pound ground beef

1/3 cup chopped onion

1/3 cup chopped celery

2 garlic cloves, minced

14 slices French bread (1/2 inch thick)

4 large tomatoes, sliced 1/2 inch thick

1 teaspoon dried basil

1 teaspoon dried parsley flakes

1 teaspoon dried oregano

1 teaspoon dried rosemary, crushed

1 teaspoon garlic powder

3/4 teaspoon salt

1/2 teaspoon pepper

2 teaspoons olive oil, divided

3 tablespoons butter

3 tablespoons all-purpose flour

1-1/2 cups whole milk

1/3 cup grated Parmesan cheese

2 cups shredded mozzarella cheese

Direction

In a skillet, cook beef, onion, celery and garlic over medium heat until beef is no longer pink; drain and set aside. Toast bread; line the bottom of an ungreased 13x9-in. baking dish with 10 slices. Top with half of the meat mixture and half of the tomatoes. Combine seasonings; sprinkle half over tomatoes. Drizzle with 1 teaspoon oil. Crumble remaining bread over top. Repeat layers of meat, tomatoes, seasonings and oil. In a saucepan over medium heat, melt the butter; stir in flour until smooth. Gradually stir in milk; bring to a boil. Cook and stir until thickened and bubbly, about 2 minutes. Remove from the heat; stir in Parmesan. Pour over casserole. Top with mozzarella. Bake, uncovered, at 350 degrees for 40-45 minutes or until bubbly and cheese is golden brown.

Nutrition:

Calories: 280 calories

Total Fat: 16g

Cholesterol: 56mg

Sodium: 500mg

Total Carbohydrate: 17g

Protein: 17g

Fiber: 2g

280. Tuna Lasagna Casserole

Serving: 12
Preparation Time: 35 Minutes
Cooking Time: 55 Minutes

Ingredients

12 lasagna noodles

1 tablespoon butter

3 tablespoons all-purpose flour

1/2 cup chicken broth

1 cup milk, divided

2 cloves garlic, minced

12 soda crackers

1 pinch Italian seasoning

3 (5 ounce) cans tuna, drained

1 1/2 cups frozen mixed vegetables

1 egg white

1/4 teaspoon salt

1/2 cup grated Cheddar cheese

1/8 teaspoon black pepper

1/2 cup grated Cheddar cheese

Direction

Preheat an oven to 350 degrees F (175 degrees C). Grease a 9x13 inch baking dish.

Fill a large pot with lightly salted water and bring to a rolling boil over high heat. Once the water is boiling, stir in the lasagna, and return to a boil. Cook the pasta uncovered, stirring occasionally, until the pasta has cooked through, but is still firm to the bite, 8 to 9 minutes. Drain well in a colander set in the sink.

Melt the butter in a saucepan over medium-low heat. Whisk in the flour, and stir until the mixture becomes paste-like and light golden brown, about 5 minutes. Gradually whisk the chicken broth and 1/2 of the milk, into the flour mixture, and bring to a simmer over medium heat. Cook and stir until the mixture is thick and smooth, 10 to 15 minutes. Stir in the remaining milk and 1/2 of the minced garlic.

Place soda crackers in a resealable plastic bag. Finely crush the crackers, then add the Italian seasoning. Combine tuna, mixed vegetables, egg white, salt, 1/2 cup of Cheddar cheese, 1/4 cup of the cracker crumbs, 1/2 cup of the flour mixture, and the remaining minced garlic in a large bowl.

Spread a thin layer of the white sauce onto the prepared baking dish, followed by a layer of lasagna noodles. Spread about 1/3 of the tuna mixture over the noodles. Repeat the noodle and tuna layering three more times, topping with the remaining flour mixture. Sprinkle the pepper evenly on top of the casserole. Cover with aluminum foil.

Bake in the preheated oven for 35 minutes. Remove from the oven and top with 1/2 cup of Cheddar cheese and the remaining cracker crumbs. Change the oven setting to broil and return the casserole to the oven. Broil until lightly brown, 2 to 3 minutes.

Nutrition:

Calories: 210 calories

Total Fat: 5.7 g

Cholesterol: 24 mg

Sodium: 222 mg

Total Carbohydrate: 24 g

Protein: 15.5 g

281.   Turkey Lasagna Rollups

Serving: 4
Preparation Time: 20 Minutes
Cooking Time: 45 Minutes

Ingredients

4 lasagna noodles

6 ounces lean ground turkey

1 small onion, chopped

1 cup chopped fresh broccoli

1/4 cup water

1 cup (8 ounces) reduced-fat ricotta cheese

1 egg, lightly beaten

1 tablespoon fat-free milk

1-1/2 teaspoons minced fresh thyme or 1/2 teaspoon dried thyme

1/4 teaspoon salt

2 cups meatless spaghetti sauce, divided

1/4 cup shredded Parmesan cheese

Direction

Cook the noodles according to package directions; rinse and drain. In a nonstick skillet, cook turkey and onion over medium heat until turkey is no longer pink. Meanwhile, in a small saucepan, bring broccoli and water to a boil. Reduce heat; cover and simmer for 5 minutes or until crisp-tender; drain. Add the broccoli, ricotta, egg, milk, thyme and salt to the turkey mixture. Spread over each noodle; drizzle each with 1/4 cup spaghetti sauce. Carefully roll up jelly-roll style. Place seam side down in an 8-in. square baking dish coated with cooking spray. Drizzle with remaining spaghetti sauce. Cover and bake at 375 degrees for 45-50 minutes or until a thermometer reads 160 degrees. Sprinkle with Parmesan cheese.

Nutrition:

Calories: 347 calories

Total Fat: 13g

Cholesterol: 110mg

Sodium: 853mg

Total Carbohydrate: 33g

Protein: 23g

Fiber: 4g

282. Turkey Ravioli Lasagna

Serving: 12
Preparation Time: 30 Minutes
Cooking Time: 35 Minutes

Ingredients

1 pound ground turkey

1/2 teaspoon garlic powder

Salt and pepper to taste

1 cup grated carrots

1 cup sliced fresh mushrooms

1 tablespoon olive oil

3-1/2 cups spaghetti sauce

1 package (25 ounces) frozen cheese ravioli, cooked and drained

3 cups shredded part-skim mozzarella cheese

1/2 cup grated Parmesan cheese

Minced fresh parsley, optional

Direction

In a large skillet, cook turkey over medium heat until no longer pink; drain. Sprinkle with garlic powder, salt and pepper; set aside. In a large saucepan, cook carrots and mushrooms in oil until tender. Stir in spaghetti sauce. Spread 1/2 cup sauce in a greased 13x9-in. baking dish. Layer with half of the ravioli, spaghetti sauce mixture, turkey and cheeses. Repeat layers. Sprinkle with parsley if desired. Cover and bake at 375 degrees for 25-30 minutes or until bubbly. Uncover; bake 10 minutes longer. Let stand 15 minutes before serving.

Nutrition:

Calories:

Total Fat: g

Cholesterol: mg

Sodium: mg

Total Carbohydrate: g

Protein: g

Fiber: g

283.   Vegetable Lasagna

Serving: 6
Preparation Time: 60 Minutes
Cooking Time: 30 Minutes

Ingredients

1/4 cup olive oil

1 medium sweet red pepper, julienned

1 medium carrot, shredded

1 small onion, chopped

5 plum tomatoes, chopped

1-1/2 cups sliced fresh mushrooms

1 small yellow summer squash, cut into 1/4-inch slices

1 small zucchini, cut into 1/4-inch slices

3 garlic cloves, minced

1 can (12 ounces) tomato paste

1 cup vegetable broth

2 tablespoons brown sugar

2 teaspoons dried oregano

2 teaspoons dried basil

1 teaspoon salt

1/2 teaspoon dried thyme

1/4 teaspoon pepper

6 lasagna noodles

1 large egg, lightly beaten

1 cup ricotta cheese

1 cup shredded part-skim mozzarella cheese

1/3 cup shredded Parmesan cheese

2 teaspoons Italian seasoning

Direction

In a Dutch oven, heat oil over medium-high heat. Add red pepper, carrot and onion; cook and stir until crisp-tender. Add tomatoes, mushrooms, yellow squash, zucchini and garlic; cook and stir until squashes are crisp-tender. Stir in tomato paste, broth, brown sugar and seasonings. Bring to a boil. Reduce heat; simmer, uncovered, 30 minutes, stirring occasionally. Meanwhile, cook noodles according to package directions; drain. Preheat oven to 350 degrees. In a small bowl, mix egg and ricotta cheese. Spread 1 cup vegetable mixture into a greased 8-in. square baking dish. Layer with two noodles (trim to fit pan), half of the ricotta mixture, about 1-1/2 cups vegetable mixture and two additional noodles. Top with remaining ricotta mixture, noodles and vegetable mixture. Sprinkle with cheeses and Italian seasoning. Bake, uncovered, 30-35 minutes or until bubbly and cheese is melted. Let stand 5 minutes before serving.

Nutrition:

Calories: 432 calories

Total Fat: 19g

Cholesterol: 68mg

Sodium: 857mg

Total Carbohydrate: 48g

Protein: 20g

Fiber: 7g

284.   Vegetarian Lasagna Loaf

Serving: 4
Preparation Time: 20 Minutes
Cooking Time: 30 Minutes

Ingredients

5 no-cook lasagna noodles

2 envelopes (1-1/4 ounces each) white sauce mix

1 tablespoon Italian seasoning

1 teaspoon garlic powder

3 cups fat-free milk

1 cup fat-free ricotta cheese

1 cup frozen California-blend vegetables, thawed

1/2 cup nonfat Parmesan cheese topping

2 tablespoons reduced-fat sour cream

1/2 cup seeded chopped fresh tomato

Direction

Break the noodles in half widthwise; set aside. In a saucepan, combine sauce mix, Italian seasoning and garlic powder. Gradually stir in milk. Bring to a boil; cook and stir for 2 minutes or until thickened and bubbly. In an 8x4-in. loaf pan coated with cooking spray, layer 1/2 cup sauce, two noodle pieces, 1/4 cup ricotta cheese, 1/4 cup vegetables and about 1-1/2 tablespoons Parmesan cheese topping. Repeat layers three times. Top with remaining noodles, sour cream, 1/2 cup sauce, tomato and remaining Parmesan cheese topping. Bake, uncovered, at 350 degrees for 30-35 minutes or until bubbly and noodles are tender. Let stand 10 minutes before serving. Reheat remaining sauce; serve with lasagna.

Nutrition:

Calories: 378 calories

Total Fat: 8g

Cholesterol: 18mg

Sodium: 1211mg

Total Carbohydrate: 52g

Protein: 24g

Fiber: 3g

285.   Weeknight Lazy Lasagna

Serving: 6
Preparation Time: 20 Minutes
Cooking Time: 10 Minutes

Ingredients

8 ounces uncooked lasagna noodles, broken into 2-inch pieces

1 cup part-skim ricotta cheese

1 cup shredded part-skim mozzarella cheese, divided

1/3 cup grated Parmesan cheese

1 jar (24 ounces) pasta sauce with meat

Direction

Preheat oven to 400 degrees. Cook lasagna noodles according to package directions. Meanwhile, in a large bowl, mix ricotta cheese, 1/2 cup mozzarella cheese and Parmesan cheese. Drain noodles well; stir into cheese mixture. Spread 1 cup pasta sauce into a greased 11x7-in. baking dish. Layer with half of the noodle mixture and 1 cup sauce; layer with the remaining noodle mixture and sauce. Sprinkle with remaining cheese. Cover with greased foil; bake until heated through, 10-15 minutes.

Nutrition:

Calories: 332 calories

Total Fat: 10g

Cholesterol: 29mg

Sodium: 901mg

Total Carbohydrate: 45g

Protein: 17g

Fiber: 3g

286.   Weeknight Ravioli Lasagna

Serving: 6
Preparation Time: 15 Minutes
Cooking Time: 45 Minutes

Ingredients

1 jar (24 ounces) pasta sauce

1 package (25 ounces) frozen meat or cheese ravioli

1-1/2 cups shredded part-skim mozzarella cheese

3 cups fresh baby spinach

Direction

Preheat oven to 350 degrees. In a small saucepan, heat sauce 5-7 minutes over medium heat or just until simmering, stirring occasionally. Spread 1/2 cup sauce into a greased 11x7-in. baking dish. Layer with half of the ravioli, 1-1/2 cups spinach, 1/2 cup cheese and half of the remaining sauce; repeat layers. Sprinkle with remaining cheese. Bake, uncovered, 45-50 minutes or until edges are bubbly and cheese is melted. Let stand 5 minutes before serving.

Nutrition:

Calories: 344 calories

Total Fat: 10g

Cholesterol: 26mg

Sodium: 850mg

Total Carbohydrate: 45g

Protein: 17g

Fiber: 5g

287.   Wheres The Squash Lasagna

Serving: 12
Preparation Time: 40 Minutes
Cooking Time: 60 Minutes

Ingredients

1 pound ground beef

2 large zucchini (about 1 pound), shredded

3/4 cup chopped onion

2 garlic cloves, minced

1 can (14-1/2 ounces) stewed tomatoes

2 cups water

1 can (12 ounces) tomato paste

1 tablespoon minced fresh parsley

1-1/2 teaspoons salt

1 teaspoon sugar

1/2 teaspoon dried oregano

1/2 teaspoon pepper

9 lasagna noodles, cooked, rinsed and drained

1 carton (15 ounces) ricotta cheese

2 cups shredded part-skim mozzarella cheese

1 cup grated Parmesan cheese

Direction

In a skillet, cook the beef, zucchini and onion over medium heat until meat is no longer pink. Add garlic; cook 1 minute longer. Drain. Place tomatoes in a food processor or blender; cover and process until smooth. Stir into beef mixture. Add the water, tomato paste, parsley and seasonings. Bring to a boil. Reduce heat; simmer, uncovered, for 30 minutes, stirring occasionally. Spread 1 cup meat sauce in a greased 13x9-in. baking dish. Arrange three noodles over sauce. Spread with a third of the meat sauce; top with half of the ricotta cheese. Sprinkle with a third of the mozzarella and Parmesan cheeses. Repeat. Top with remaining noodles, meat sauce and cheeses.

Cover and bake at 350 degrees for 45 minutes. Uncover; bake 15 minutes longer or until bubbly. Let stand for 15 minutes before cutting.

Nutrition:

Calories: 309 calories

Total Fat: 13g

Cholesterol: 53mg

Sodium: 642mg

Total Carbohydrate: 27g

Protein: 21g

Fiber: 3g

288.   White Lasagna

Serving: 8-10
Preparation Time: 25 Minutes
Cooking Time: 35 Minutes

Ingredients
9 lasagna noodles
1/4 cup butter, cubed
1/3 cup all-purpose flour
1 tablespoon minced dried onion
1/4 teaspoon garlic powder
1/8 teaspoon pepper
2 cups chicken or turkey broth
1 cup milk
1 cup grated Parmesan or Romano cheese, divided
1 can (4 ounces) sliced mushrooms, drained
1 package (10 ounces) frozen cut asparagus or 3/4 pound fresh cut asparagus, cooked and drained
2 cups cubed cooked chicken or turkey
1 package (6 ounces) sliced or shredded mozzarella cheese
6 ounces thinly sliced cooked ham, chopped
Direction
Cook noodles according to package directions. Drain. In a large saucepan, melt butter; blend in flour, onion, garlic powder and pepper. Add broth and milk; cook and stir until bubbly and thickened. Stir in 1/2 cup Parmesan cheese. Spread 1/2 cup sauce in the bottom of a greased 13x9-in. baking pan. Stir mushrooms into the remaining sauce. Lay 3 noodles in the pan. Top with asparagus, chicken, mozzarella and about 1 cup sauce. Top with 3 more noodles, the cooked ham and half of the remaining sauce. Cover with remaining noodles and sauce. Sprinkle with the remaining Parmesan cheese. Bake, uncovered, at 350 degrees for 35 minutes or until heated through.
Nutrition:
Calories: 322 calories
Total Fat: 15g
Cholesterol: 66mg
Sodium: 678mg
Total Carbohydrate: 25g
Protein: 24g
Fiber: 2g

289.   White Sauce Lasagna

Serving: 14-16
Preparation Time: 25 Minutes
Cooking Time: 30 Minutes

Ingredients

1 pound ground beef

1 cup finely chopped celery

1 cup finely chopped onion

1 garlic clove, minced

1 cup half-and-half cream

3 ounces cream cheese, cubed

2 teaspoons dried basil

1 teaspoon dried oregano

1/2 teaspoon Italian seasoning

1/2 teaspoon salt

1/2 teaspoon pepper

2 cups shredded cheddar cheese

7 ounces shredded Gouda cheese

2 cups (16 ounces) 4% cottage cheese

1 large egg, lightly beaten

8 ounces lasagna noodles, cooked and drained

12 ounces sliced or 3 cups shredded part-skim mozzarella cheese

Minced fresh parsley

Direction

In a large skillet, cook the beef, celery and onion over medium heat until
meat is no longer pink. Add garlic. Cook for 1 minute or until garlic is
tender; drain. Stir in the cream, cream cheese, basil, oregano, Italian
seasoning, salt and pepper; cook and stir over low heat until blended.
Gradually add cheddar and Gouda cheeses, stirring until cheese is melted;
remove from heat. Combine cottage cheese and egg; set aside. Layer half of
the lasagna noodles in a greased 13x9-in. baking dish. Top with half of the

meat sauce, half of the cottage cheese mixture and half of the mozzarella cheese. Repeat layers with remaining ingredients. Bake at 375 degrees, uncovered, for 30-35 minutes. Sprinkle with parsley. Let stand for 10 minutes before serving.

Nutrition:

Calories: 329 calories

Total Fat: 19g

Cholesterol: 87mg

Sodium: 526mg

Total Carbohydrate: 15g

Protein: 24g

Fiber: 1g

290.   Ziti Lasagna

Serving: 3
Preparation Time: 15 Minutes
Cooking Time: 20 Minutes

Ingredients

2 cups uncooked ziti or small tube pasta

1/2 pound lean ground beef

1/4 cup chopped onion

1/4 cup chopped green pepper

1 can (8 ounces) tomato sauce

1/2 teaspoon Italian seasoning

1/4 teaspoon garlic powder

Dash pepper

3/4 cup ricotta cheese

1 cup shredded part-skim mozzarella cheese

Direction

Cook ziti according to package directions. Meanwhile, in a skillet, cook the beef, onion and green pepper over medium heat until meat is no longer pink; drain. Stir in the tomato sauce, Italian seasoning, garlic powder and pepper. Cook and stir until heated through, about 3 minutes. Drain pasta. Spread half of the meat sauce in a 1-qt. baking dish coated with cooking spray. Top with half of the ziti, ricotta cheese and mozzarella cheese. Repeat layers. Bake, uncovered, at 350 degrees for 20-25 minutes or until heated through. Let stand for 5 minutes before serving.

Nutrition:

Calories: 437 calories

Total Fat: 15g

Cholesterol: 83mg

Sodium: 613mg

Total Carbohydrate: 38g

Protein: 35g

Fiber: 2g

291. Zucchini Beef Lasagna

Serving: 12
Preparation Time: 50 Minutes
Cooking Time: 30 Minutes

Ingredients
1 pound lean ground beef (90% lean)
2 garlic cloves, minced
2 cans (8 ounces each) no-salt-added tomato sauce
1/2 cup water
1 can (6 ounces) tomato paste
2 bay leaves
1 teaspoon minced fresh parsley
1 teaspoon Italian seasoning
1 package (16 ounces) lasagna noodles, cooked, rinsed and drained
1 cup (8 ounces) fat-free cottage cheese
1 small zucchini, sliced and cooked
1 cup (8 ounces) reduced-fat sour cream
Direction
In a large skillet, cook beef and garlic over medium heat until meat is no longer pink; drain. Add the tomato sauce, water, tomato paste, bay leaves, parsley and Italian seasoning. Bring to a boil; reduce heat. Simmer, uncovered, for 30-40 minutes. Discard bay leaves. Spread 1/2 cup meat sauce in a 13-in. x 9-in. baking dish coated with cooking spray. Arrange five noodles over sauce, cutting to fit. Spread with cottage cheese. Cover with five noodles, half of the meat sauce and the zucchini. Cover with five noodles and sour cream. Top with remaining noodles and meat sauce. Bake, uncovered, at 350 degrees for 30-35 minutes or until heated through. Let stand for 15 minutes before cutting.
Nutrition:
Calories: 187 calories
Total Fat: 8g
Cholesterol: 21mg
Sodium: 270mg
Total Carbohydrate: 19g
Protein: 14g
Fiber: 2g

292.   Zucchini Red Pepper Lasagna

Serving: 12
Preparation Time: 20 Minutes
Cooking Time: 55 Minutes

Ingredients

1 carton (15 ounces) ricotta cheese

1-1/2 cups shredded part-skim mozzarella cheese, divided

2 large eggs

3 tablespoons prepared pesto

2 cups sliced zucchini

2 cups sliced baby portobello mushrooms

2 tablespoons canola oil

2 jars (one 24 ounces, one 14 ounces) meatless spaghetti sauce

9 no-cook lasagna noodles

1 jar (12 ounces) roasted sweet red peppers, drained and chopped

Direction

In a small bowl, combine the ricotta cheese, 1/2 cup mozzarella cheese, eggs and pesto; set aside. In a large skillet, sauté zucchini and mushrooms in oil until tender; set aside. Spread 1 cup spaghetti sauce in a 13x9-in. baking dish coated with cooking spray. Top with three noodles; spread 1 cup sauce to edges of noodles. Layer with half of the zucchini mixture, red peppers and cheese mixture. Top with three more noodles and another cup of sauce. Layer with remaining zucchini mixture, peppers, cheese mixture, noodles and sauce. Cover and bake at 375 degrees for 45 minutes or until a thermometer reads 160 degrees. Uncover; sprinkle with remaining mozzarella cheese. Bake 10 minutes longer or until cheese is melted. Let stand for 15 minutes before cutting.

Nutrition:

Calories: 241 calories

Total Fat: 11g

Cholesterol: 59mg

Sodium: 651mg

Total Carbohydrate: 23g

Protein: 13g

Fiber: 3g

293.　Cheesy Egg Noodles

Servings: 4

Ingredients:

1/2 cup cream cheese, softened

5-1/2 tbsp mozzarella cheese, freshly grated

5 tbsp + 2 tsp parmesan cheese, freshly grated

3 egg yolks

1/8 tsp garlic powder

1/8 tsp black pepper, ground

1/2 tsp Italian seasoning

Directions:

Preheat the oven to 475 degrees F.

In a large bowl, beat the egg yolks together with cream cheese. Add in mozzarella and parmesan and continue beating with a hand mixer.

Add all the remaining ingredients. Mix until thoroughly combined.

Transfer the mixture to a baking pan lined with parchment paper. Flatten batter using the back of a spoon or a spatula.

Place the baking pan in the oven and then lower the temperature to 350 degrees F. Bake for about 5 minutes. If you see small bubbles forming, lower the temperature to 300 degrees F and keep baking for another 2 minutes or until the center and all sides are done.

Remove pan from oven and allow to cool for 15 minutes at room temperature. Slice baked pasta to 1/2- to 1/4-inch strips using a pizza cutter or sharp knife. Serve noodles topped with some low-carb sauce.

294.   Egg Noodles With Mayo

Servings: 2

Ingredients:

3 eggs, large

2 tbsp cream cheese, softened

2 tsp psyllium husk powder

1 tbsp mayo

1/4 tsp salt

Directions:

Preheat the oven 350 degrees F.

Place all the ingredients in a blender. Blend on high until dough becomes smooth. Allow dough to rest for at least 10 minutes before proceeding to the next step.

Transfer dough onto a baking pan lined with a silicone mat or parchment paper. Spread evenly using a flat plastic spatula.

Bake dough for 8 to 10 minutes. Slowly peel dough from mat. If it still sticks, bake for a few more minutes.

Remove baked dough from oven and set aside for 15 minutes to cool

Peel the dough from silicone mat or parchment paper. Using a sharp knife, cut pasta into 1/4-inch wide strips. Serve pasta with your favorite sauce.

295.   Carnivore Egg Noodles

Servings: 2

Ingredients:

3 eggs, large

1 tbsp cream cheese, softened

3 tbsp pork rinds, finely ground

1 tbsp dry parmesan cheese, grated

Directions:

Preheat the oven 350 degrees F.

Place all the ingredients in a blender. Blend on high until dough becomes smooth.

Transfer dough onto a baking pan lined with silicone mat or parchment paper. Spread evenly using a flat plastic spatula.

Bake for 8 to 10 minutes. Try peeling dough from mat. If it still sticks, bake for a few more minutes.

Remove baked dough from the oven and set aside for 15 minutes to cool.

Peel dough from silicone mat or parchment paper. Cut pasta into 1/4-inch wide strips using a sharp knife. Serve with your choice of sauce.

296.　Lasagna Sheets

Servings: 3

Ingredients:

1/2 cup + 2 tbsp cream cheese, softened

4 large eggs, beaten

2-1/2 tbsp psyllium husk powder

1/2 tsp salt

Directions:

Preheat the oven to 300 degrees F.

Combine cream cheese, eggs, and salt in a medium sized mixing bowl. Whisk until mixture becomes a smooth batter.

Slowly whisk in psyllium husk. Mix until fully incorporated. Set aside batter for a few minutes.

Place batter between two sheets of parchment paper. Using a rolling pin, flatten batter according to your desired thickness of pasta. If you want thinner lasagna sheets, prepare lasagna in two equal batches.

Transfer pasta onto a baking pan, including the bottom parchment paper. Bake for 10 to 12 minutes. Remove from oven and set aside to cool.

Peel off the parchment paper. Using a pizza cutter or sharp knife, slice lasagna into sheets depending on the size of your baking dish.

297.   Two Cheese Lasagna

Servings: 4

Ingredients:

1-1/2 cups mozzarella cheese, shredded

1/2 cup cream cheese, softened

2 eggs, large

1 tbsp basil, chopped

1 tsp baking powder

1 tsp garlic powder

Directions:

Preheat oven to 350 degrees F.

Place all the ingredients in a food processor. Pulse until mixture achieves a smooth and thick consistency.

Transfer the batter into a baking pan lined with parchment paper. Flatten and spread the batter evenly using a plastic spatula or the back of a spoon.

Bake for about 25 minutes. Make sure not to overbake lasagna. Remove from oven and set aside to cool.

Once cooled, slice lasagna into sheets that will fit your baking dish. To cook, layer with your prepared filling and bake for 25 minutes in an oven preheated to 375 degrees F.

298.   Three Cheese Lasagna Sheets

Servings: 4

Ingredients:

1/2 cup cream cheese, softened

1-1/4 cup whole milk mozzarella cheese, shredded

1/4 cup parmesan cheese, grated

2 eggs, large

1/4 tsp garlic powder

1/4 tsp onion powder

1/4 tsp Italian seasoning

Directions:

Preheat the oven to 375 degrees F.

Place the eggs and cream cheese in a large bowl and mix them together using a hand mixer. Add all the other ingredients except for mozzarella cheese. Mix until fully combined.

Fold in the mozzarella cheese using a rubber spatula. Mix until the cheese is fully incorporated.

Transfer the batter onto a 9x13 baking pan lined with parchment paper. Flatten the batter, making sure that it forms an even layer and covers the whole pan.

Bake for 20 to 25 minutes on the middle rack. Once done, place lasagna sheets in the fridge to cool.

After about 20 minutes, cut lasagna into thirds. These will be perfect for an 8.5 x 4.5 x 2.5 pan.

299.   Chicken Lasagna Noodles

Servings: 5

Ingredients:

1 lb ground chicken

1/3 cup parmesan cheese, shredded

1/3 cup full-fat mozzarella cheese

1 egg, large

1 tsp Italian seasoning

1/4 tsp salt

pinch of ground black pepper

Directions:

Preheat oven to 400 degrees F.

Combine all the ingredients in a large mixing bowl. Mix thoroughly and form into a ball.

Transfer dough to a baking pan lined with parchment paper. Roll out ball and flatten into a thin and even layer. Make sure to cover the bottom of the pan completely.

Bake for about 10 minutes or until lasagna noodle is firm. Remove from oven and slice into sheets that will fit your dish.

To cook, bake prepared lasagna for 15 minutes in an oven preheated to 400 degrees F.

300. Beef Lasagna Noodles

Servings: 5

Ingredients:

1 lb ground beef, lean

1/4 cup parmesan cheese, grated

1/2 egg yolk, lightly beaten

1/2 tbsp Italian seasoning

1/2 tsp onion powder

1/2 tsp garlic powder

salt and pepper, to taste

Directions:

Preheat oven to 450 degrees F.

In a small bowl, mix together the Italian seasoning, onion powder, garlic, salt, and pepper.

Place beef in a large mixing bowl and add the mixed dry ingredients. Mix well.

Add the egg yolk and parmesan. Mix until all ingredients are fully incorporated.

Transfer mixture into a baking pan lined with parchment paper. Flatten and spread the mixture evenly, making sure that the pans are covered from edge to edge. If layer is too thick, use an additional baking pan.

Bake for 7 to 12 minutes. When "noodles" are just browned, remove from oven. Drain any grease. Slice baked noodles to fit your lasagna dish.

To cook, bake prepared lasagna for 15 minutes in an oven preheated to 400 degrees F.

301.   Lasagna With Coconut Flour

Servings: 5

Ingredients:

8 eggs, large

1/2 cup + 1 tbsp cream cheese, softened

3 tbsp coconut flour

1-1/4 tbsp psyllium husk powder

1 tsp xanthan gum

1 tsp salt

Directions:

Preheat oven to 320 degrees F. Line 2 baking pans with parchment paper.

Add salt to cream cheese and then manually whisk in eggs one by one. Don't use an electric mixer.

Combine coconut flour, psyllium husk, and xanthan gum in a separate bowl. Mix thoroughly.

Add dry ingredients to eggs and cheese mix. Whisk vigorously by hand or with an electric whisk until batter is smooth. Allow to rest and thicken for a minute.

Divide the batter evenly between the 2 baking pans. Quickly spread the batter out as you pour, making sure it evenly covers the whole pan and is very thin.

Bake for 10 to 13 minutes or until edges have begun to shrink and top has become opaque. Try to peel off parchment paper. If it still sticks, bake for a few more minutes. If not, remove from oven and allow to cool.

Once cooled, remove parchment paper and allow pasta to air dry. After a couple of hours, cut into the size you need.

302.   Soy Pasta

Servings: 4

Ingredients:

1/2 cup full-fat soy flour

1/2 cup protein powder + extra for dusting

1 egg, large

1/4 tsp garlic powder

1/4 tsp salt

1/2 cup water

Directions:

Mix together soy flour, protein powder, garlic powder, and salt. Whisk in egg, and then add water. Continue mixing until all ingredients are fully incorporated and a sticky dough is formed.

Sprinkle some protein powder on your work surface. Divide dough into 2 equal portions. Dust each portion liberally with protein powder and using a rolling pin, roll out and flatten dough into a very thin layer.

Cut the dough into 1/8- to 1/4-inch wide strips using a sharp knife or a pizza cutter. Place pasta strips on parchment paper and air dry for 2 hours.

To cook, place the noodles in boiling salted water for 1 to 2 minutes.

303. Manicotti With Coconut Flour

Servings: 8

Ingredients:

3/4 cup cream cheese, softened

1/3 cup parmesan cheese, grated

6 eggs, large

1-1/2 tbsp coconut flour

1/8 tsp xanthan gum

1 tbsp butter

Directions:

Place the cream cheese, parmesan, and eggs in a blender. With the blender set on low, blend until ingredients are completely mixed.

While the blender is still running, add the coconut flour and xanthan gum. Continue blending until batter is thick. Scrape the sides and blend on medium setting for a few seconds. Allow batter to rest for a few minutes.

Place a non-stick pan over low heat. To make pasta, brush the pan with lightly with butter. Pour about 1/4 cup of batter into the center of the pan. Spread batter into a disc by tilting the pan in a circular motion. Cook for 1-2 minutes or until set and the edge browns. Using a spatula greased with butter, carefully flip the pasta. After 15 to 20 seconds, remove pasta from the pan.

Do the same with the remaining batter. You should be able to make 8 to 10 pieces.

Assemble manicotti by placing your prepared filling in each piece and rolling up into a log tightly.

To cook, place manicotti seam-side down in a lightly greased baking dish with your pasta sauce. Cover the dish with cling film and microwave for about 5 minutes.

304. Ravioli

Servings: 6

Ingredients:

1 cup blanched almond flour

1/4 cup coconut flour

1 egg, large and lightly beaten

2 tsp xanthan gum

2 tsp apple cider vinegar

5 tsp water

1/4 tsp salt

Directions:

Place coconut flour, almond flour, xanthan gum, and salt in a food processor. Pulse until ingredients are thoroughly mixed.

Add apple cider vinegar while processor is running followed by the egg. Continue pulsing while adding 1 tsp of water at a time. Use water as needed to make dough that is firm but still feels sticky and without creases.

Wrap dough in cling film and knead a few minutes. Set aside for 15 minutes to rest and place in the fridge. Leave dough in the fridge for at least 45 minutes and up to 5 days.

Divide dough evenly into several portions. Roll out and flatten each portion of dough. They should be thin enough to roll through your pasta machine.

Press dough between parchment paper to make sure it won't fall apart. Roll each flattened dough through the largest setting of your machine. Fold the dough over and roll through the machine again using the same setting.

Continue rolling dough through smaller settings until dough becomes approximately 1/16-inch thick and translucent against natural light.

You can now add your prepared filling to the pasta. Once you're done, put ravioli on a baking pan. Freeze for 15 minutes before cooking.

To cook, pan fry for 1 to 2 minutes on each side or boil in salted water for 3 to 5 minutes.

305. Spätzle

Serving: 2

Ingredients:

2 eggs, large

1/2 cup oat fiber

1/4 cup glucomannan powder

2 tbsp baking powder

2 tbsp wheat gluten

1 tsp salt

1-1/2 cup hot water

Directions:

Place the oat fiber, glucomannan powder, baking powder, wheat gluten, and salt in a mixing bowl. Mix until ingredients are fully combined.

Heat the water in the microwave for 1 minute.

Add the egg and water to the dry mixture. Whisk quickly and vigorously until you form a dough that's not too sticky and that can be shaped into a ball.

Transfer dough onto a parchment paper or a smooth surface. Set aside for about 5 minutes to rest.

Divide the dough into small balls. Add each ball into your extruder or noodle press to form the noodles. Place noodles on a parchment paper and allow to rest for 8 to 10 minutes.

To cook, place pasta in boiling water for 1 minute or less. Transfer cooked pasta into cold water and drain.

Conclusion

Pasta has travelled a lot in time and space and from the very first steps made towards this meant the beginning of a new era in gastronomy. Nowadays, pasta is eaten all over the world, in its many variations. From the Far East to the Middle East and to the American Western Coast and from the Northern countries to New Zealand and Australia, everybody is familiar with pasta. And the best part about it is that everybody loves it. There are so many types of pasta, pasta sauces, pasta shapes and pasta recipes in general that it is impossible not to find at least one recipes you will deeply fall in love with.

And they are all easy to make, even for beginners.

The next step is to get into the kitchen and allow yourself to be creative. Remember that pasta is a dish that was born out of poverty and that people needed to be creative when it came to their dishes. This means that although the recipes presented in this book are incredibly delicious, you are always allowed to make tour own combinations.

Allow yourself to be creative. Allow yourself to make the combinations that will amaze, that will surprise and that will satisfy those who will eat them. The power to create new dishes is in your hands! Open your mind because pasta can really go well with almost anything out there, from mushrooms and veggies to cheese to all types of meat and fish.